STEM CELLS - LABORATORY AND CLINICAL RESEARCH

GENETIC AND EPIGENETIC ALTERATIONS THAT DRIVE LEUKEMIC STEM CELL SELF-RENEWAL

STEM CELLS - LABORATORY AND CLINICAL RESEARCH

Additional books in this series can be found on Nova's website under the Series tab.

Additional E-books in this series can be found on Nova's website under the E-books tab.

STEM CELLS - LABORATORY AND CLINICAL RESEARCH

GENETIC AND EPIGENETIC ALTERATIONS THAT DRIVE LEUKEMIC STEM CELL SELF-RENEWAL

JAN JACOB SCHURINGA
VINCENT VAN DEN BOOM
AND
SARAH J. HORTON

Novinka
Nova Biomedical Books
New York

Copyright © 2010 by Nova Science Publishers, Inc.

All rights reserved. No part of this book may be reproduced, stored in a retrieval system or transmitted in any form or by any means: electronic, electrostatic, magnetic, tape, mechanical photocopying, recording or otherwise without the written permission of the Publisher.

For permission to use material from this book please contact us:
Telephone 631-231-7269; Fax 631-231-8175
Web Site: http://www.novapublishers.com

NOTICE TO THE READER
The Publisher has taken reasonable care in the preparation of this book, but makes no expressed or implied warranty of any kind and assumes no responsibility for any errors or omissions. No liability is assumed for incidental or consequential damages in connection with or arising out of information contained in this book. The Publisher shall not be liable for any special, consequential, or exemplary damages resulting, in whole or in part, from the readers' use of, or reliance upon, this material.
Independent verification should be sought for any data, advice or recommendations contained in this book. In addition, no responsibility is assumed by the publisher for any injury and/or damage to persons or property arising from any methods, products, instructions, ideas or otherwise contained in this publication.
This publication is designed to provide accurate and authoritative information with regard to the subject matter covered herein. It is sold with the clear understanding that the Publisher is not engaged in rendering legal or any other professional services. If legal or any other expert assistance is required, the services of a competent person should be sought. FROM A DECLARATION OF PARTICIPANTS JOINTLY ADOPTED BY A COMMITTEE OF THE AMERICAN BAR ASSOCIATION AND A COMMITTEE OF PUBLISHERS.

Library of Congress Cataloging-in-Publication Data

Available upon Request
ISBN: 978-1-61728-379-6

Published by Nova Science Publishers, Inc. ✝ New York

Contents

Preface		vii
Introduction		1
Chapter I	Genetic Alterations in LSCs that Affect Self-renewal and/or Differentiation	3
Chapter II	Epigenetic Alterations in LSCs that Affect Self-renewal and/or Differentiation	17
Chapter III	Multiple (EPI) Genetic Defects Are Required for Leukemic Transformation	27
Chapter IV	Conclusions	31
References		33
Index		53

Preface

Acute myeloid leukemia has emerged as a paradigm for the concept of the cancer stem cell. This hypothesis presumes that the disease is maintained by a rare population of leukemia-initiating stem cells which have acquired genetic or epigenetic changes. It is most likely that a single (epi)genetic event will not be sufficient to cause leukemia, but that a number of sequential events are required. Similar to normal hematopoietic stem cells, both intrinsic as well as extrinsic factors that arise from the bone marrow niche, provide essential cues that regulate cell fate decisions such as leukemic stem cell self-renewal and differentiation. In this chapter, we will review the genetic and epigenetic abnormalities that underlie the process of leukemic transformation, and will discuss which events potentially co-operate to induce leukemia.

Introduction

Acute myeloid leukemia (AML) arises from genetic defects in the hematopoietic stem cell (HSC). HSCs can undergo self-renewal divisions to ensure maintenance of the stem cell pool as well as generate large numbers of mature functional blood cells via migration, differentiation, proliferation and (anti-) apoptotic events. Complex processes such as self-renewal and differentiation must be tightly controlled as a shift in the balance towards self-renewal severely impairs the hematopoietic process and might ultimately lead to the development of AML [1]. Thus a thorough understanding of the mechanisms involved in the regulation of self-renewal divisions of normal and leukemic stem cells are pivotal in tackling the highly malignant disorder of AML.

AML is in most cases a stem cell disease [2-4]. The malignant clone is hierarchically organized – strikingly similar to the normal hematopoietic system [5]- and consists of rare leukemic stem cells (LSC) that have the exclusive capacity to transfer disease into irradiated recipients. The more committed blast population within the leukemic clone lacks these properties. The most convincing evidence comes from transplantation studies in which the SCID leukemia-initiating cells (SL-IC) of all subtypes of AML, regardless of the heterogeneity in maturation characteristics of the leukemic blasts, resided exclusively in the immature $CD34^+/CD38^-$ compartment [2,4]. However, this finding was challenged recently by a study which demonstrated that most SL-ICs were present in the $CD34^+/CD38^+$ fraction of AML samples when the immune mediated clearance of anti-CD38 coated cells was prevented [6]. Thus a multipotent progenitor (MPP) rather than an HSC may serve as the cell of origin in some AMLs and this will be discussed in more detail in part I.

Leukemic transformation is regarded as a multistep process in which a number of sequential events ultimately induce the full spectrum of leukemia [7,8]. These transformation steps include chromosomal translocations such as t(8;21), inv(16) and t(15;17), as well as mutations in tyrosine kinase receptors (FLT3, C-KIT) or signal transduction molecules such as RAS, JAK2 and NPM1 (reviewed in [8,9]). Multiple events ultimately lead to enhanced self-renewal and differentiation defects of the LSC. A number of studies have indeed elegantly shown that oncogenes such as AML1-ETO and FLT3-ITDs do not result in leukemic transformation individually, but act synergistically when expressed within the same stem cell [7]. Furthermore, the fact that the incidence of AML increases with age (approximately half of AML patients are more than 65 years of age) further strengthens the notion that an accumulation of genetic and/or epigenetic alterations makes the stem cell compartment more prone to the development of AML. In this chapter we will review the current understanding of how genetic and epigenetic events might affect stem cell self-renewal properties and how these hits might collaborate in the process of leukemic transformation.

Chapter I

Genetic Alterations in LSCs that Affect Self-renewal and/or Differentiation

I-I. Translocations

CBF Fusion Genes

The genes encoding the heterodimeric transcription factor complex AML1/CBFβ are among the most frequently mutated in human acute leukemia. CBFβ enhances the DNA binding capacity of AML1, whose target genes play critical roles in hematopoiesis. Conditional gene targeting studies in mice have demonstrated that while both subunits are essential for fetal HSC development, CBFβ but not AML1 is essential for the maintenance of adult HSCs [10]. The most common chromosomal rearrangements involving the *AML1/CBFβ* genes are the t(8;21)(q22;q22) translocation which generates the *AML1-ETO* fusion gene and inv(16)(p13q22) which generates the *CBFβ-MYH11* fusion gene. Various mouse models have been generated in an attempt to model disease induced by these fusion proteins. A myeloproliferative disorder resulted when AML1-ETO expression was targeted to the HSC compartment using the *SCA1* promoter (Table 1, [11]). However, other

AML1-ETO models did not result in the development of AML unless the animals were treated with mutagenic agents [12].

Although AML1-ETO conditional knock-in mice did not develop AML, myeloid progenitors isolated from these mice displayed enhanced re-plating potential *in vitro* [13]. Furthermore, elevated numbers of HSCs and abnormal myeloid cells were observed in the bone marrow of mice transplanted with AML1-ETO retrovirally transduced murine HSCs [14]. Retroviral delivery of AML1-ETO to human $CD34^+$ cord blood cells resulted in HSC expansion in stromal co-culture assays and enhanced proliferation in cytokine driven liquid cultures. However, transplantation of these cultured cells into NOD/SCID mice did not result in leukemia [15-17]. Taken together these studies suggest that AML1-ETO expression promotes the self-renewal of HSCs but requires co-operating mutations to induce overt leukemia.

The mechanisms by which AML1-ETO promotes the self-renewal of HSCs remain unclear although up-regulation of survivin expression may be a contributing factor [18]. The finding that the *AML1-ETO* translocation can be detected in neonatal Guthrie card spots suggests that the translocation occurs *in utero* as the initiating event and results in the generation of a pre-leukemic clone. Secondary genetic or epigenetic events are then required for the development of clinically overt leukemia [19]. A recent report found that AML1-ETO expressing cells displayed an enhanced mutation rate *in vivo* and suggested that AML1-ETO may directly facilitate the acquisition of secondary events by suppressing endogenous DNA repair pathways [20].

In contrast to AML1-ETO, CBFβ-MYH11 conditional knock-in mice spontaneously developed AML in the absence of mutagen treatment [21]. Interestingly the genes *Plag1* or *Plag2*, which were previously shown to co-operate with CBFβ-MYH11 in AML development [22], were over-expressed in many of the AML samples in this conditional model. Retroviral over-expression of CBFβ-MYH11 increased the proliferative capacity of human $CD34^+$ CB cells but did not result in leukemia upon transplantation into NOD/SCID mice [23]. These studies suggest that like AML1-ETO, expression of CBFβ-MYH11 confers a pre-leukemic status to the cells by enhancing their self-renewal. Subsequent alterations which will be discussed later on are required for the transition to overt leukemia.

RARα Fusion Genes

The promyelocytic leukemia – retinoic acid receptor alpha (PML-RARα) fusion protein, which is expressed as a result of the t(15;17)(q22;q21) translocation, is found in > 95% of cases of acute promyelocytic leukemia (APL).

Table 1. Summary of the models for the most common genetic events in myeloid leukemia

Translocations			
Gene	Model	Phenotype	Ref.
AML1-ETO	Mouse Transgenic-*Sca1*	Myeloproliferative disorder.	[11]
	Mouse Knock-in	Embryonic lethal. Abnormal myeloid cells in fetal liver with increased self-renewal potential.	[194]
	Mouse Conditional knock-in	Enhanced re-plating *in vitro*. AML upon ENU treatment.	[13]
	Mouse Retroviral transduction	Increased numbers of abnormal cells in the BM. No AML.	[14]
	Human (CD34$^+$ CB) Retroviral transduction	Long-term proliferation *in vitro*. No AML.	[15,17]
CBFβ-SMMHC	Mouse Knock-in	Embryonic lethal. Lack of definitive hematopoiesis.	[195]
	Mouse Knock-in chimera	Block in myeloid and lymphoid differentiation. AML after ENU treatment.	[196]
	Mouse Conditional knock-in	AML with median latency of 5 months.	[21]
	Human (CD34+ CB) Retroviral transduction	Increased proliferation *in vitro*. No leukemia.	[23]
PML-RARα	Mouse Transgenic- *hCathepsin G*	Myeloproliferative disorder, low frequency of APL with long latency.	[26,27]
	Mouse Transgenic- *hMRP8*	Low frequency of APL with long latency.	[25]
	Mouse Transgenic – *hCD11b*	Slight impairment in hematopoiesis. No leukemia.	[28]
	Mouse (lin⁻ BM) Retroviral transduction	Short latency, high penetrance APL. Impaired neutrophil differentiation.	[30]

Table 1 (Continued)

	Human (lin⁻ PB) Retroviral transduction	Enhanced promyelocytic differentiation but subsequent block in vitro.	[29]
NUP98-Hoxa9	Mouse Transgenic - hCathepsin G	Myeloproliferative disorder, eventual progression to AML.	[197]
	Mouse (whole BM) Retroviral transduction	Myeloproliferative disorder, eventual progression to AML.	[35]
	Human (CD34⁺ CB) Retroviral transduction	Increased proliferation and HSC self-renewal *in vitro* and *in vivo*.	[36]
MLL-AF9	Mouse Knock-in	AML within 6-9 months preceded by myeloproliferation. Small number of ALL cases.	[198,199]
	Mouse (cKit⁺ BM) Retroviral transduction	Myeloid immortalisation *in vitro*, AML *in vivo*.	[42]
	Human (Lin⁻ CB) Retroviral transduction	Enhanced proliferation *in vitro*. ALL upon transplantation into NOD/SCID mice.	[43]
	Human (CD34⁺ CB) Retroviral transduction	Immortalisation *in vitro*. AML or ALL *in vivo*.	[44]
MLL-ENL	Mouse Translocator	Rapid AML within 4 months.	[48]
	Mouse (Lin⁻ BM) Retroviral transduction	Myeloid immortalisation *in vitro*, AML *in vivo*.	[41]
	Human (Lin⁻ CB) Retroviral transduction	Enhanced proliferation in vitro. ALL in NOD/SCID mice.	[43]
BCR-ABL (p210)	**Mouse Transgenic - *metallothionein***	T, B or myeloid acute leukemia	[200,201]
	Mouse Transgenic - *Tec*	ALL in founder mice. CML in transgenic progeny.	[202]
	Mouse Transgenic inducible (Tet-Off system)	Acute pre-B cell leukemia reversible upon tetracycline treatment.	[203]
	Mouse Transgenic-*Sca1*	CML with longer latency (4-18 months). Progression to either myeloid or lymphoid blast crisis.	[59]
	Mouse (whole BM) Retroviral transduction	CML with short latency and high penetrance. T lymphoid lymphoma or CML in secondarys.	[56,57]
	Human (Lin⁻ CB) Retroviral transduction	Enhanced erythroid differentiation *in vitro*,	[58,204]

		myeloproliferative disease *in vivo*.	
	Point mutations / insertions		
CEBPα	**Mouse** N-terminal knock-in mutant (p42 deficient)	AML with complete penetrance. Latency 6 months – 1 year.	[74]
	Mouse Knock-in mutant chimeras	C-terminal mutant: Immature erythroid leukemia.	[75]
		N-terminal mutant: AML with shorter latency than C-terminal.	
		Combined mutants: AML with shorter latency than either mutant alone.	
	Mouse (Lin- BM) Retroviral transduction N-terminal mutant	Altered kinetics but no differentiation block *in vitro*.	[205]
	Human (CD34+ CB) Retroviral transduction N-terminal mutant	Block in differentiation at abnormal promyelocytic stage *in vitro*.	[205]
FLT3-ITD	**Mouse** Knock-in	Fatal myeloproliferative disorder. Median latency 10 months.	[82]
	Mouse (BM) Retroviral transduction	Lethal myeloproliferative disorder. Latency 40 – 60 days.	[81]
	Human (CD34⁺ CB) Retroviral transduction	Enhanced proliferation and self-renewal *in vitro*.	[83]
Flt3-TKD	**Mouse (BM)** Retroviral transduction	Lymphoid disease with long latency. T cell lymphoma or B-ALL.	[88]
cKit^{V814}	**Mouse** Transgenic – $H\text{-}2L^d$	ALL or lymphoma in 4/15 mice.	[89]
	Mouse (BM) Retroviral transduction.	Factor-independent growth *in vitro*. Lymphoid leukemia *in vivo*. Latency 6-19 weeks.	[89]
NPMc⁺	**Mouse** Transgenic – *hMRP8*	Non-fatal myeloproliferative disease from 6 months of age.	[93]
Kras^{G12D}	**Mouse** Conditional Knock-in	Fatal myeloproliferative disorder with complete penetrance.	[99]
	Mouse – Conditional knock-in. BM chimeras.	T cell malignancies and JMML depending on cell dosage used.	[103]
Kras^{G12D}	**Mouse (BM)** Retroviral transduction	CMML. Median latency 64 days.	[97]
Nras^{G12D}	**Mouse (BM)** Retroviral transduction	AML (latency 49.5 days) or CMML (latency 62.5 days).	[97]
NRAS^{G13C}	**Human (CD34⁺ CB)** Retroviral transduction	Enhanced myeloid proliferation and monocytic differentiation *in vitro* and *in vivo*.	[98]

This theory is supported by the lack of PML-RARα expression in the HSC ($CD34^+CD38^-$) compartment isolated from APL patients [24] and the inability of these cells to transplant leukemia into NOD/SCID mice [2].

Transgenic mice in which PML-RARα expression was driven from promoters expressed during the myeloid- promyelocytic stages of differentiation (*Cathepsin G* and *MRP8*), developed APL after long latency and low penetrance [25-27]. In contrast, mice in which PML-RARα expression was directed from a promoter expressed at a later stage of myeloid differentiation (*CD11b*), did not develop leukemia [28]. These studies highlight the importance of proper targeting of PML-RARα expression. The hMRP8-PML-RARα transgenic mice displayed a pre-leukemic phase which was associated with impaired neutrophil differentiation [25]. Impaired differentiation was also observed upon retroviral delivery of PML-RARα expression to both murine and human hematopoietic stem and progenitor cells (HSPCs) [29,30]. In contrast to the transgenic mice, the murine transduction/transplantation model gave rise to short latency APL with high penetrance. It is possible that retroviral insertional mutagenesis rapidly met the requirement for co-operating mutations in this model. Alternatively, the targeting of PML-RARα expression to more primitive hematopoietic progenitor cells rather than committed myeloid cells may explain the difference in penetrance and latencies.

The mechanism underlying the differentiation block induced by PML-RARα has been the subject of intense investigations. Both wild-type retinoic acid receptor (RARα) and PML-RARα mediate the transcriptional repression of retinoic acid (RA) target genes by binding the nuclear co-repressors NCOR and SMRT which recruit histone deacetylases (HDACs) – these are described in more detail in part II. During normal myeloid differentiation, physiological concentrations of retinoic acid (RA) induce the dissociation of the co-repressors and associated HDACs from RARα allowing the recruitment of transcriptional activators and normal myeloid differentiation. However, physiological concentrations of RA do not permit the dissociation of co-repressors and HDACs from the PML-RARα complex thus resulting in a block in differentiation [31]. This block is alleviated by higher concentrations of RA which is used in the clinic in combination with chemotherapy to achieve remission in the majority of patients.

Many AML cells exhibit enhanced survival upon genotoxic stress yet do not carry mutations of the *p53* tumour suppressor gene. In many cases the leukemic cells have acquired more subtle ways to inhibit p53 function. For example, the PML-RARα fusion protein retains the ability to interact with the product of the remaining wild-type *PML* allele which normally associates with p53. Recruitment of p53 to the PML-RARα/HDAC complex results in the inhibition of p53 acetylation and subsequent inactivation [32]. An alternative mechanism is proposed for AMLs with the t(8;21) translocation in which AML1-ETO has been shown to directly repress transcription of the p53 checkpoint mediator *p14ARF* [33].

NUP98 Fusion Genes

The *NUP98* gene undergoes reciprocal chromosomal translocations with many other partner genes and is hence one of the most promiscuous fusion partner genes in leukemia. *NUP98*-fusion genes are found in patients with AML, myelodysplastic syndrome, or blast crisis CML [34]. The *NUP98* nucleoporin gene encodes an important component of the nuclear pore complex. To date 21 fusion partners of NUP98 have been described of which the most common and extensively studied is NUP98-Hoxa9. Retroviral transduction of murine HSPCs with NUP98-HOXA9 enhanced the proliferation of myeloid progenitors *in vitro* and induced a myeloproliferative disorder *in vivo* which eventually progressed to AML. The latency of AML progression was markedly decreased upon co-expression of MEIS1 which also co-operates with wild-type HOXA9 to induce AML [35]. Retroviral transduction of human CD34$^+$ cells with NUP98-HOXA9 enhanced HSC proliferation and expansion *in vitro* and *in vivo*. Impaired neutrophil differentiation in response to G-CSF was also observed [36]. Gene expression profiling revealed that the Hox genes *Hoxa7*, *Hoxa9* and their co-factor *Meis1*, well recognized for their ability to induce AML in animal models [37], were up-regulated upon NUP98-HOXA9 expression in both murine and human models [36,38]. Several genes including *CEBPα* were also down-regulated upon NUP98-HOXA9 expression in human CD34$^+$ cells. Interestingly, restoration of *CEBPα* expression impaired the proliferation of NUP98-HOXA9 transduced cells suggesting that down-modulation of *CEBPα* expression by this fusion protein contributes to enhanced HSC proliferation and impaired differentiation [36]. A recent study using a transgenic Notch reporter mouse very elegantly demonstrated that NUP98-HOXA9 enhanced HSC self-renewal by increasing the number of HSCs undergoing symmetrical cell divisions. In contrast, the *BCR-ABL* fusion gene promoted proliferation but did not alter the ratio of symmetric versus asymmetric cell division [39].

MLL Fusion Genes

Like many of the genes involved in chromosomal translocations in acute leukemia, MLL plays an important role in normal hematopoietic development and is essential for definitive hematopoiesis [40]. Over 50 fusion partner genes of *MLL* have been identified so far of which the most common are *AF9*, *ENL* and *AF4*. Immortalized myeloid cell lines were efficiently generated following retroviral transduction of murine HSPCs with either MLL-ENL or MLL-AF9. Retrovirally transduced cells were able to induce AML with short latency and high penetrance upon transfer into mice [41,42]. Both fusion proteins were also able to enhance the proliferation of human cord blood cells and induce ALL upon transplantation into NOD/SCID mice [43]. However, the skew towards ALL in this model did not faithfully recapitulate the disease in humans. In patients the *MLL-ENL* fusion gene is found in both acute myeloid and lymphoid leukemia, while *MLL-AF9* is primarily associated with myeloid leukemia. Another study using human cord blood cells demonstrated that MLL-AF9 was able to give rise to either AML or ALL and this depended on the recipient strain of mice. AML was observed if the cells were transplanted into NOD/SCID-SGM3 (which are engineered to produce human SCF, GM-SCF and IL3) and ALL was observed if the mice were transplanted into NOD/SCID/$\beta 2m^{-/-}$ mice [44]. These results suggest that the microenvironment plays an important role in the lineage of the leukemia.

Retroviral delivery of MLL-ENL to purified populations of murine HSCs, committed myeloid progenitors (CMPs) or granulocyte-macrophage progenitors (GMPs) followed by transplantation into recipient mice resulted in AML from all three populations [45]. This study demonstrated that MLL-fusions are able to impose self-renewal activity on committed progenitors which normally lack this ability. Using an MLL-AF9 retroviral transduction/transplantation model LSCs were identified which shared the same phenotype as the GMP from which they arose and expressed a self-renewal signature normally only observed in HSCs [46]. However, a recent study using MLL-AF9 'knock-in' mice in which MLL-AF9 expression was directed from the endogenous *MLL* promoter revealed that physiological levels of MLL-AF9 expression were not sufficient to transform GMPs [47].

The inter-chromosomal recombination model is perhaps the most elegant model to study the role of chromosomal translocations in leukemia. Gene targeting in mice was used to engineer *loxP* sites into the murine *MLL* and *ENL* loci. When these mice were crossed with *Lmo2-Cre* mice, the *de novo* translocation of *MLL* and *ENL* loci occurred specifically in hematopoietic cells and resulted in the generation of both reciprocal translocation products. The resultant MLL-ENL translocator mice developed AML rapidly within 4 months of birth suggesting that secondary alterations are not required in this model [48].

The models described above indicate that MLL-fusions promote the proliferation and self-renewal of hematopoietic progenitor cells. The mechanisms by which MLL-fusion proteins transform cells remain elusive although *HOX* genes and their associated co-factors play an important role. Multiple *HOXA* genes, the HOX co-factors *MEIS1* and *PBX3* and *FLT3* are up-regulated in patients with MLL translocations [49]. Several studies have shown that both wild-type MLL and MLL-fusion proteins directly regulate the expression of a subset of 5'*HoxA* genes [50-52]. Recent studies have shown that both HOXA9 and MEIS1 are required for the maintenance of immortalisation by MLL-fusion proteins and loss of expression of either gene induces growth arrest, apoptosis or differentiation of leukemic or immortalised cells [53-55].

BCR-ABL

The p210 BCR-ABL fusion protein is expressed as a result of the t(9;22)(q34;q11) chromosomal translocation. This translocation is found in the vast majority of CML patients and results in the generation of a constitutively active tyrosine kinase. Many murine retroviral transduction/transplantation models have been described which model the human disease with variable efficiency. Most of the studies demonstrated that BCR-ABL expression was sufficient to induce CML with a very short latency in recipient mice [56,57]. However, these studies were not very efficient at modeling the progression to myeloid blast crisis, which is eventually observed in CML patients if left untreated. Retroviral transduction of human Lin⁻ cord blood cells with BCR-ABL resulted in enhanced erythroid differentiation *in vitro* and a low incidence of myeloproliferative disease upon transplantation into NOD/SCID/$\beta 2m^{-/-}$ mice [58]. Targeting of BCR-ABL expression to the HSC compartment using the Sca1 promoter resulted in the most faithful model of CML so far although in this model BCR-ABL expression was limited to HSCs and was not expressed in more mature cells [59]. These mice developed CML with relatively long latency which progressed to either myeloid or lymphoid blast crisis. The CML cells from these mice displayed genomic instability as previously reported in CML patient samples [60]. Interestingly, the CML was reversible upon elimination of LSCs thus providing proof that elimination of LSCs is of therapeutic benefit [59].

It is assumed that transition to blast crisis is associated with the acquisition of secondary events. In support of this, activation of the Wnt signaling pathway through increased nuclear localization of β-catenin was observed in patients with accelerated phase and blast crisis CML. Furthermore, activation of the Wnt pathway endowed granulocyte-macrophage progenitors (GMPs) isolated from CML patients with self-renewal activity [61]. Although there are multiple lines of evidence to suggest that CML arises as a result of BCR-ABL expression in an HSC [62,63], this data suggests that during disease progression to blast crisis the LSC may evolve from an HSC to a GMP as a result of secondary genetic or epigenetic events. The study outlined previously by Wu et al showed that BCR-ABL acts to enhance proliferation rather than self-renewal of HSCs. Several studies showed that the Stat5 transcription factor is an important mediator of this effect [64-67]. In addition to STAT5, BCR-ABL is known to regulate several other signaling networks including RAS, ERK and CRKL [68]. In addition, RAC and Hedgehog signaling play an important part in leukemogenesis mediated by BCR-ABL. BCR-ABL hyper-activates RAC1 and RAC2 and both genes are required for BCR-ABL induced CML in mouse models [69]. Loss of

Smoothened, an important component of the Hedgehog pathway also impairs CML induction by BCR-ABL [70].

I-II. Point Mutations/Insertions

CEBPα

AML patients without detectable chromosomal aberrations often harbor point mutations or insertions/deletions involving *CEBPα*, *FLT3*, *cKIT* or *NPM*. CEBPα is a transcription factor required for the CMP-GMP transition in normal hematopoiesis [71]. It is translated into two major polypeptides of 42 kDa (p42) and 30 kDa (p30) due to alternative translation initiation. Two major groups of *CEBPα* mutations are observed in AML; N-terminal and C-terminal mutations. Leukemic cells often possess mutations in both alleles of *CEBPα*; 1 allele harbors an N-terminal mutation and the other a C-terminal mutation [72]. Homozygous N- or C- terminal mutations are almost never observed in AML suggesting that there is selection for both types of mutation during leukemic progression. N-terminal mutations cause a frame shift leading to loss of the p42 isoform whereas C-terminal mutations involve insertions/deletions within the DNA binding domain of CEBPα [73]. The N-terminal mutation was very elegantly modeled by engineering the mouse *Cebp* locus to only express the p30 isoform. These mice uniformly developed AML within 1 year of birth. Interestingly, committed myeloid cells were capable of transferring disease to secondary recipients in this model implying that the CEBPα mutant confers self-renewal to this population [74]. The *Cebp* locus was also modified such that only the C-terminal CEBPα mutation was expressed. Since *CEBPα* mutations often result in embryonic lethality the combined effects of both N- and C-terminal mutations were studied in chimeric mice. Mice engrafted with fetal liver cells expressing only the C-terminal CEBPα mutation displayed an expansion of pre-malignant HSCs and developed leukemia which had an immature erythroid phenotype and a longer latency than chimeric mice expressing only the N-terminal mutation. Chimeric mice engrafted with cells expressing both N- and C-terminal mutations developed AML more rapidly than mice expressing either mutation alone suggesting that these mutations co-operate in AML progression [75]. Other mutations also result in the de-regulation of CEBPα function. The NUP98-HOXA9 and AML1-ETO fusion proteins down-regulate its expression [36,76]. Also PML-RARα can bind to CEBPα and prevent it from binding to its target gene promoters [77]. Therefore, alterations in CEBPα function may be a very common event in leukemogenesis and are thought to contribute to the differentiation block observed in AML.

FLT3 and cKIT

Mutations resulting in constitutive activation of receptor tyrosine kinases are frequently observed in AML. The FLT3 and cKIT receptors are normally activated by the ligands FLT3L and SCF respectively and are required for the survival, proliferation and normal differentiation of HSPCs [78,79]. *FLT3*-internal tandem duplications (ITDs) are frequently found in AML patients and are associated with a particularly poor prognosis. Point mutations in the tyrosine kinase domain (TKD) of *FLT3* are less common in AML. They are often observed in pediatric ALL patients with *MLL*-rearrangements and T-ALL [80]. Several models have provided insight into the role of these activated kinases in leukemia. Over-expression of FLT3-ITD in murine HSPCs resulted in a lethal myeloproliferative disorder when transplanted into mice [81]. The same outcome was observed when FLT3-ITD expression was directed from the endogenous *Flt3* promoter using a knock-in approach [82]. Retroviral delivery of FLT3-ITD to human $CD34^+$ cord blood cells resulted in enhanced progenitor self-renewal, proliferation and erythroid differentiation [83]. These effects were not observed upon over-expression of wild-type FLT3 in these models. This may be because FLT3-ITD, but not wild-type FLT3, is able to activate STAT5 [84] and several studies have demonstrated that this transcription factor is a critical mediator of FLT3-ITD activity. Co-expression of a dominant-negative STAT5 mutant in human cord blood cells abrogated FLT3-ITD-induced progenitor proliferation [83]. Furthermore, mice which expressed a mutated FLT3-ITD incapable of activating Stat5 failed to develop myeloproliferative disease (MPD) [85]. FLT3-ITD not only enhances proliferation but also survival of leukemic cells by up-regulating the expression of MCL1 and SURVIVIN [86,87].

Interestingly, FLT3-TKD mutants are much less effective at activating STAT5 and also display a distinct biology to FLT3-ITD mutants. Whereas mice expressing FLT3-ITD developed MPD, mice expressing FLT3-TKD developed lymphoid disorders (T cell lymphoma or B-ALL) instead [88]. A similar phenotype was observed upon over-expression of the cKIT^{V814} mutant in murine HSPCs. This mutant conferred growth factor independence to these cells and induced lymphoid leukemia with incomplete penetrance when transplanted into mice [89]. The lack of AML in these models suggests that by themselves these mutations are not sufficient to transform the myeloid lineage and require co-operating mutations to do so. This is consistent with the finding that *cKIT* mutations are frequently observed in AML patients expressing the *AML1-ETO* or *CBFβ-MYH11* fusion genes [90].

NPM

Mutations of the *Nucleophosmin1* gene (*NPM1*) occur in approximately 60% of AML cases with normal karyotype. NPM normally shuttles between the nucleus and the cytoplasm to fulfill its role in centrosome duplication and ribosome biogenesis. All NPM1 mutations lead to common alterations of the C-terminus, which result in exclusive cytoplasmic localization of the mutant (NPMc$^+$) protein [91]. Transformation assays have demonstrated that NPMc$^+$ behaves as an oncogene and antagonizes the tumor suppressor function of ARF [92]. Recently a transgenic mouse model was reported in which expression of NPMc$^+$ was directed from the human *MRP8* promoter. Although these mice developed a myeloproliferative disorder, they did not progress to AML [93].

RAS

Oncogenic *NRAS* and *KRAS* point mutations have been identified in myeloid and T cell disorders. Aberrant RAS signaling is particularly prevalent in juvenile myelomonocytic leukemia (JMML) [94]. RAS proteins are small GTPases which normally cycle between an active

GTP-bound state and an inactive GDP-bound state. Activating *RAS* mutations prevent the hydrolysis of RAS-GTP and result in constitutive activation of the protein [95]. RAS proteins play a role in regulating multiple processes including proliferation, differentiation and survival [96]. Various models have successfully recapitulated the disorders associated with these mutations in humans. Murine HSPCs over-expressing $KRAS^{G12D}$ or $NRAS^{G12D}$ gave rise to CMML or AML upon transplantation into mice [97]. $NRAS^{G12D}$ over-expression in human $CD34^+$ cord blood cells enhanced proliferation and monocytic differentiation but did not induce disease in NOD/SCID mice [98]. Conditional expression of the $KRAS^{G12D}$ mutant from the endogenous *Ras* promoter resulted in a lethal myeloproliferative disease with complete penetrance [99,100]. The disease was found to originate from the HSC compartment in which elevated levels of pSTAT5, pERK and pS6 were induced by $KRAS^{G12D}$ [101]. Due to possible non cell-autonomous effects in this model, bone marrow cells conditionally expressing $KRAS^{G12D}$ from the endogenous promoter were used in competitive transplantation assays. Recipient mice developed T-cell leukemia, T cell lymphoma or a disease resembling JMML. Limiting dilution experiments revealed that the *Kras* mutation was insufficient for frank malignancy and co-operating events were acquired during the course of the experiment [102,103]. In addition to direct mutation of the *RAS* genes, the RAS signaling pathway is activated by a variety of other mechanisms including mutation of the *NF1* or *PTPN11* genes which regulate RAS-GTP levels but also by the BCR-ABL fusion protein [104] and mutant FLT3 [105].

Chapter II

Epigenetic Alterations in LSCs that Affect Self-renewal and/or Differentiation

Apart from genetic alterations acting as one of the steps in development of leukemia, epigenetic events have gained much interest for their role in leukemogenesis. The term epigenetics was coined by Sir Conrad Hall Waddington in 1942 but its definition in biology has been revisited and was recently described as: "an epigenetic trait is a stably heritable phenotype resulting from changes in a chromosome without alteration in the DNA sequence" [106,107]. This means that the phenotypical outcome of a genotype is not static, but can be modified by epigenetic processes. Epigenetic regulation of gene expression is regulated at the chromatin level. Microscopically, in interphase cell nuclei two types of chromatin can be observed: condensed chromatin (heterochromatin) and open chromatin (euchromatin). Heterochromatin is associated with silent genes whereas euchromatin contains mainly actively transcribed genes. The regulation of the chromatin structure is orchestrated at the level of the nucleosome, the structural unit of chromatin. A nucleosome is comprised of 146 bp DNA wrapped around a histone octamer, containing four different histones (H2A, H2B, H3 and H4) all present in duplicate. The amino-termini of the histones are unstructured and protrude from the nucleosomal core structure. These can be chemically altered by specific histone-modifying enzymes at various residues in several ways (acetylation, methylation, hosphorylation, ubiquitination etc.) [108]. Different modifications are involved in inducing either open or condensed chromatin. For example, acetylated histones are found in active chromatin and acetyl groups can be added to histones by histone acetyl transferases (HATs) and removed by histone deacetylases (HDACs). Histone methylation is present in both active and repressed chromatin, depending on the residue that is modified in the histone tail. DNA methylation is another well-known epigenetic modification which directly targets the genomic DNA. In mammals, cytosine residues in the context of CpG dinucleotides can be methylated by DNA methyltransferases (DNMTs). Methylation of CpG-dense regions (CpG islands, CGIs) in the promoters of genes causes repression of the transcriptional activity. Mechanistically, DNA methylation can act in two different ways. First, CpG methylation can interfere with the binding of activating transcription factors to CpG-containing sequences. Secondly, methylated CpGs can be targeted by methyl-CpG-binding proteins (i.e. MBDs), which can recruit HDACs resulting in deacetylation of genes that are targeted by DNA methylases [109,110]. In normal cells only a small fraction of the CGIs are methylated and the majority (~85%) are hypomethylated. In contrast, outside promoter regions and CGIs the genomic DNA is globally hypermethylated [111,112]. Data from multiple model organisms suggest a role for intra- and intergenic DNA methylation in maintenance of genome integrity, silencing of transposons and inhibition of cryptic transcription initiation.

Aberrant Epigenetic Regulation in AML

Given the fact that epigenetic regulation can induce a stable heritable gene expression profile in cells, a role for epigenetic events in generation and clonal expansion of cancer cells is very likely. Increasing knowledge about aberrant epigenetic activation of oncogenes and/or silencing of tumor suppressor genes underlines the importance of epigenetic events in tumor formation. Here we will discuss the role of abnormal epigenetic regulation in the process of leukemogenesis and more specifically in acute myeloid leukemia (AML). We will discuss important epigenetic pathways affected in AML and how this might contribute to development and progression of the disease.

DNA Methylation

DNA methylation was the first epigenetic modification found to be dramatically changed in cancer cells. Despite a reduction in global methylation levels in cancer cells, promoter-specific hypermethylation is observed. Together, this leads to unwanted transcription of repeats, activation of genes and abnormal silencing of tumor suppressor genes [113]. Inactivation of tumor suppressors is known to provide a major contribution to cancerous growth of cells and is suggested to take place in the initial steps of cancer development [114]. These tumor-suppressor genes are referred to as "epigenetic gatekeepers" and a classical example, which is commonly hypermethylated in various types of solid tumors, is the *p16INK4A* gene. Down-regulation of the p16INK4A transcript is known to result in increased self-renewal of stem cells and progenitors allowing more time for cells to develop secondary genetic abnormalities like mutations or translocations. In AML, *p16INK4A* hypermethylation is observed less frequently. In contrast, AML and myelodysplastic syndrome (MDS) patients often display hypermethylation of *p15INK4B*, a gene located directly upstream of *p16INK4A* in the genome [115-118]. p15INK4B is highly homologous to p16INK4A and most likely plays an important role in hematopoietic cell lineages. AML patients in clinical remission with a methylated *p15INK4B* show an increased risk of relapse and a significant reduction in survival [119]. Although *p15Ink4B*$^{-/-}$ mouse models do not spontaneously develop myeloid leukemias, they do display extramedullary hematopoiesis and lymphoid hyperplasia in the spleen and reactive lymph nodes [120]. Furthermore, heterozygous deletion of *p15Ink4B* increases the frequency of retrovirus-induced myeloid leukemia in mice [121]. Apart from *p15INK4B* other frequently hypermethylated genes in AML include, among others, *CALCITONIN*, *E-CADHERIN*, *ER* and *MDR1*. Genome-wide analyses of DNA hypermethylation in AML patients at diagnosis and relapse showed an increase in DNA methylation at relapse, indicating that in myeloid malignancies DNA hypermethylation is not only involved in the initiation of disease but also during disease progression [122]. Very recently, genome-wide DNA methylation profiles of 344 AML patients were generated [123]. Clustering analysis identified 16 groups with distinct methylation profiles. Some of these groups correlated with known mutations (*CEBPα*) or translocations (*e.g. AML-ETO* and *PML-*

RARα). Interestingly, 5 groups did not correlate with a specific genetic abnormality but did predict clinical outcome, underlining the biological and clinical relevance of these DNA methylation profiles in AML. Clinical intervention in aberrant DNA hypermethylation became possible with the approval of 5-azacytidine and 5-aza-2'-deoxycytidine (decitabine), which induce global hypomethylation. Decatibine treatment of MDS patients induces re-expression of the p15INK4B transcript and critically improved the survival of MDS patients [124,125].

Histone Acetylation

Histone acetylation is a chromatin mark associated with actively transcribed genes. Several lysine residues on the tails of histone H3 and H4 can be acetylated by histone acetyl transferases (HATs). The identified HATs can be categorized in three different families: GCN5/PCAF, MYST and p300/CBP. Within the MYST family, two members have been reported to be translocated in AML: MOZ (MYST3) and MORF (MYST4). Many different translocations producing *MOZ* fusions have been identified, including t(8;16)(p11;p13) [126] resulting in *MOZ-CBP* and t(8;22)(p11;q13) [127,128], inv(8)(p11;q13) [129,130] and t(8; 20)(p11;q13) [131] generating *MOZ-p300*, *MOZ-TIF2* and *MOZ-NcoA3* respectively. For the *MORF* gene only the t(10;16)(q22;p13) translocation has been identified which generates a *MORF-p300* fusion [132,133]. It is proposed that expression of these fusions leads to aberrant histone acetylation, thereby inducing leukemogenesis. Interestingly, HAT activity was dispensable for leukemic transformation by MOZ-TIF2 in mouse bone marrow transplants [134]. However, it was shown that MOZ-TIF2 expression leads to aberrant recruitment of CBP and p300 to target genes of nuclear receptors and p53 [135,136]. Gene targeting studies in mice revealed that MOZ is very important for maintenance of the HSC pool during early hematopoiesis and important for proper reconstitution of recipient mice in transplantation experiments [128,137]. Mice carrying a single point mutation in the HAT catalytic domain also display reduced numbers of HSCs and progenitors underlining the importance of HAT activity in normal hematopoiesis [138]. Gene expression analysis of AML patients with the *MOZ-CBP* t(8;16)(p11;p13) translocation showed increased expression of *HOXA9*, *HOXA10* and *MEIS1* [139]. Over-expression of these genes has been associated with leukemogenesis [37]. Up-regulation of *HOX* genes by MOZ-CBP does not reflect aberrant targeting of the fusion product since the wild-type MOZ protein is known to regulate *HOX* gene expression during development, but rather is a result of deregulation of HAT activity of the fusion protein [140-142].

Histone Methylation

Histone methylation is a chromatin modification that is found on both active and silent genes. Depending on the specific residue being methylated the mark poises activation or repression of a gene. A large group of highly conserved methyltransferases has been identified that target lysine or arginine residues on amino-termini of histone H3 and H4 [108]. The specificity of methyltransferases is much higher than that of histone acetyl transferases and in general they are specific for a single residue. In addition, residues can be either mono-, di- or tri-methylated, which cause different outcomes in terms of gene regulatory activity. In this chapter we will focus on two specific types of histone methylation, which are both involved in tumor formation and progression, despite their opposing activities in modulating gene activity.

H3K4 Methylation

A classical histone methyltransferase gene affected in leukemia is *Mixed Lineage Leukemia* (*MLL*). A number of translocations generating *MLL* fusions have been introduced in this chapter already. The *MLL* gene was initially identified as a member of the Trithorax family of transcriptional activators in *Drosophila* [143]. The Su(var)3-9, Enhancer-of-zeste, Trithorax (SET) domain at the C-terminus of MLL possesses methyltransferase activity specific for lysine 4 on histone H3 (H3K4), a modification associated with transcriptional activation. Wild-type MLL resides in a multi-protein complex which regulates the maintenance, but not the initiation of *HOX* gene expression during early development [51,144]. Since *Mll* knockout mice are embryonic lethal, much attention has been directed to the role of *Mll* in fetal hematopoiesis. $Mll^{-/-}$ mice display defects in HSC maintenance and progenitor differentiation, which is at least in part dependent on correct expression of *Hox* genes, since re-expression of some *HOX* genes (*HOXA9*, *HOXA10* and *HOXB4*) can revert the progenitor phenotype [40,145,146]. Conditional *Mll*-null models revealed that MLL plays an important role in adult hematopoiesis since it is required to maintain the quiescence of the HSC pool [147,148].

Interestingly, MLL fusion proteins all lack a functional SET domain, since the part of the *MLL* gene encoding the SET domain is lost in the fusion gene [149]. However, they are still targeted to genes regulated by wild-type MLL and induce their aberrant activation. [50-52]. This activation is likely due to the fact that at least a set of MLL fusion proteins (*i.e.* MLL-ENL, MLL-AF4 and MLL-AF10) are capable of recruiting the non-SET domain containing histone methyltranferase DOT1L, which can methylate histone H3 at lysine 79 (H3K79), a modification associated with active transcription [150,151]. In addition, genome-wide analysis of MLL-AF4 induced histone modification patterns in a cell line model showed a dramatically changed chromatin interaction profile at target genes compared to wild-type MLL, which also likely contributes to aberrant gene expression [152]. The interaction between MLL fusions and DOT1L takes place via the ENL, AF4 or AF10 moiety of the fusion. This may imply that H3K79 methylation renders MLL target genes active (*e.g. HOX* genes), even in the absence of a functional MLL SET domain, thereby compensating for the loss of MLL H3K4 methyltransferase activity.

Although for a long time histone methylation was thought of as a stable epigenetic mark, the identification of a large family of histone demethylases showed that regulation of histone methylation is much more dynamic [153]. Recently, a translocation, t(11;21;12)(p15;p13;p13), was identified in AML patients generating a NUP98-JARID1A fusion, the latter being a H3K4 demethylase [154]. The fusion encodes the C-terminus of JARID1A, which contains a plant homeodomain (PHD) motif, which is known to 'read' the histone code and can bind di- and tri-methylated H3K4. Mice transplanted with retrovirally transduced lineage-negative bone marrow cells over-expressing the fusion protein quickly developed leukemia, which was dependent on the functionality of the PHD motif [155]. The authors show that NUP98-JARID1A prevents demethylation of H3K4 thereby interfering with down-regulation of transcription factors during lineage-commitment, including the *Hox* genes, *Meis1* and *Pbx1*. Taken together these data underline the importance of correct regulation of H3K4 methylation in prevention of leukemogenesis.

H3K27 Methylation

H3K4 methylation-dependent activation of transcription by the Trithorax family of transcriptional activators (including MLL) is counteracted by the Polycomb group family of transcriptional repressors, which were first identified in *Drosophila*, and are responsible for silencing the expression of many developmental genes [143,156]. The Polycomb group proteins are found in different multi-protein complexes, which together operate in initiating and maintaining silencing of their target genes. The complex believed to initiate Polycomb-mediated repression is the Polycomb repressive complex 2 (PRC2), consisting of the core components EZH2, EED, SUZ12 and RbAp46/48. EZH2 was found to be a SET-domain containing histone methyltransferase specific for lysine 27 on histone H3 (H3K27) [157]. Methylation of H3K27 is thought to be the initiating event in Polycomb silencing. PRC1, another Polycomb repressive complex consisting of RING1A/B, HPC, HPH, BMI1 and SCMH can recognize trimethylated H3K27 though the HPC protein [158]. PRC1 recruitment to promoters was shown to block chromatin remodeling and prevent initiation, but not binding, of RNA polymerase II [159,160]. The RING1 subunit of the PRC1 is capable of ubiquitinating lysine 119 at histone H2A (H2AK119) [161,162]. To what extent ubiquitination of H2AK119 is a key process in Polycomb-mediated silencing is not completely resolved. $Bmi1^{-/-}$ mice display loss of H2A ubiquitination at almost 700 gene promoters and leads to their increased expression (*i.e. Hox* genes), suggesting that H2A ubiquitination is important for Polycomb silencing [163,164]. Genome-wide localization analysis of PRC components have shown that not all Polycomb target genes are bound by both PRC1 and PRC2 complexes, indicating the existence of multiple modes of Polycomb-mediated repression [165-167].

Both the PRC1 and PRC2 complexes have been linked to tumor formation. A role for *EZH2* in cancer was suggested from work on both prostate and breast tumors showing over-expression of EZH2 correlates with a poor prognosis [168-170]. AML cell survival was shown to be significantly impaired when cells were treated with an EZH2 inhibitor, indicating that also in AML cells EZH2 plays an important role in disease progression. In addition, EZH2 over-expression prevents HSC exhaustion in a murine transplantation models, indicating that the protein is involved in dealing with replicative stress in HSPCs [171]. In the specific case of *PML-RARα* translocations, it was shown that EZH2 can be recruited by the fusion protein and represses its target genes, thereby contributing to the leukemogenic phenotype [172]

Another Polycomb group protein whose high expression correlates with poor prognosis in AML and other hematological diseases is BMI1 [173-175]. BMI1 was initially observed to be oncogenic in a retroviral integration site screen where it was identified as a collaborating hit in MMLV-induced B-cell lymphomas in Eμ-*myc* transgenic mice [176,177]. Knocking out the *Bmi1* gene results in reduced numbers of hematopoietic progenitors and more differentiated cells, eventually leading to hematopoietic failure [178]. More detailed analysis showed that BMI1 has a central regulatory role in self-renewal of HSCs by inducing symmetrical cell division both in mouse and human model systems [179-182]. Accordingly, $Bmi1^{-/-}$ mice display dramatically reduced HSC frequencies. BMI1 is also required for self-renewal of LSCs [181]. Over-expression of HOXA9 and MEIS1 in $Bmi1^{-/-}$ fetal liver cells and subsequent transplantation to irradiated recipients led to the development of AML. However, the leukemic cells could not repopulate secondary recipients suggesting that in the absence of Bmi1 the LSCs became exhausted. RNAi-mediated knockdown of BMI1 in both human cord blood and primary AML cells resulted in decreased self-renewal and led to induction of apoptosis [183]. Mechanistically, the role of BMI1 in regulating HSC self-renewal is partially explained by its ability to repress the *INK4A/ARF* locus [179,184]. Expression of p16INK4A and p19ARF in HSCs induces cell cycle arrest and p53-mediated cell death. Loss of BMI1 expression most likely results in a decreased H2AK119 ubiquitinating activity of the PRC1 complex at the *INK4A/ARF* locus, inducing expression of p16INK4A and p19ARF expression. Importantly, the hematopoietic phenotype of $Bmi1^{-/-}$ mice is not only dependent on the induction of *INK4A/ARF*. $Bmi1^{-/-}$ $Ink4A/Arf^{-/-}$ double knockout mice showed a partial recovery of hematopoietic cell counts but did not show a complete reversal of the Bmi1 null phenotype, suggesting that other pathways are also involved [185]. A candidate *INK4A/ARF*-independent pathway for BMI1 in controlling HSC and LSC self-renewal is regulation of reactive oxygen species (ROS) in the cell. Recently, it was shown that $Bmi1^{-/-}$ mice display impaired mitochondrial function due to increased expression of Polycomb target genes involved in ROS metabolism [186]. Long-term HSCs from $Bmi1^{-/-}$ mice showed increased levels of ROS and treatment of mice with the antioxidant N-acetylcysteine (NAC) resulted in a rescue of thymocyte cell numbers compared to non-treated $Bmi1^{-/-}$ mice. Furthermore, de-regulated ROS metabolism induced activation of the DNA damage response pathway. Knockout of *Chk2*, a component of the DNA damage response pathway, in $Bmi1^{-/-}$ background resulted in partial reversal of the thymocyte phenotype observed in $Bmi1^{-/-}$ mice. In addition, knockdown of BMI1 in human cord blood also induces increased ROS levels and apoptosis [187]. These data clearly show that apart from the well known role of BMI1 in regulating cell cycle and senescence through the *INK4A/ARF* locus, BMI1 is also implicated in other pathways regulating oxygen metabolism. It is clear that up-regulation of BMI1 in leukemic cells undoubtedly will give an advantage for these cells to cope with high oxygen levels. This is certainly advantageous for LSCs which are most likely not located in the oxygen-poor HSC niche and suffer from increased oxygen stress compared to normal HSCs.

Chapter III

Multiple (EPI) Genetic Defects Are Required for Leukemic Transformation

It is clear from the models summarized in part I that many if not all of the genetic events described are not sufficient to induce AML by themselves but require co-operating events to do so. The original two-step model of leukemogenesis was first proposed by Dash and Gilliland who postulated that two types of mutations (class I and class II) are required for the development of AML. Class I mutations are thought to confer a proliferative or survival advantage to the cell and class II mutations impair differentiation and enhance self-renewal. It has been generally considered that *FLT3*, *cKIT*, and *N-RAS* mutations are class I mutations and balanced translocations including *AML1/ETO*, *CBFB/MYH11*, *PML/RARA*, and *MLL* abnormalities are class II mutations [187]. This hypothesis has gained support from the findings that co-expression of various class I and class II mutations do indeed co-operate to induce leukemia in animal models. For example, the incidence of mice developing APL upon expression of PML-RARα was dramatically increased and the latency shortened following co-expression of FLT3-ITD or KRAS [188,189]. Furthermore, co-expression of FLT3-ITD and AML1-ETO, which individually are insufficient to cause disease, resulted in fatal acute leukemia [190]. These models are clinically relevant since the FLT3-ITD mutation is frequently found in patients harboring the t(8;21) or t(15;17) translocations. Activating cKIT mutations are frequently observed in patients with the t(8;21) or inv(16) translocations [90]. Consistent with this activated c-KIT co-operates with AML1-ETO to induce leukemia in a murine transduction/transplantation model [191]. The frequent co-existence of NPM1 and FLT3-ITD mutations in AML patients [192] suggests (according to the classical two-hit model) that NPM1 mutations block differentiation or enhance self-renewal.

However, as yet there is no evidence to support the idea that genetic mutations exclusively affect either the proliferation/survival (class I) or differentiation (class II). In fact, various genetic mutations often affect both of these pathways. Furthermore, many other cell biological properties of leukemic cells are frequently altered, including interactions with the bone marrow microenvironment, regulation of oxidative stress and DNA repair, and the process of self-renewal whereby the symmetry of stem cell divisions might be affected. Also, we hypothesize that leukemogenesis does not necessarily result as a consequence of two or more genetic events but may be mediated by a combination of genetic and epigenetic events.

Clearly, in some instances epigenetic changes can occur as a consequence of genetic abnormalities. Some epigenetic modifiers are directly targeted by a translocation (e.g. *MLL, MOZ, JARID1A*), which leads to aberrant epigenetic signaling. This could be due to either mistargeting of a functional epigenetic modifier (including an active catalytic domain) or correct targeting of an inactive form which blocks other chromatin modifying enzymes or sequesters other epigenetic modifiers. A classical example of the latter situation is the *MLL-AF9* translocation which leads to deregulated *HOX* gene expression due to aberrant targeting of DOT1L to its target genes [150,151]. Another example of translocations affecting the epigenetic state of genes are the PML-RARα and PLZF-RARα fusions, which are capable of recruiting the PRC2 and PRC1 complex respectively, leading to Polycomb-mediated silencing of their target genes [172,193].

On the other hand, epigenetic changes might be viewed as autonomous processes independent of genetic instability. Aging has dominant affects on the epigenetic landscape of hematopoietic stem cells, and myeloid leukemias arise particularly in elderly patients. Thus, it seems plausible that changes in epigenetic landscapes, for instance associated with aging, might contribute to the leukemic transformation process as well. The possibility to perform genome-wide analyses epigenetic landscapes has set the stage for in depth analysis of epigenetic profiles in AML patients with known translocations or normal karyotypes. The recent publication by Figuero and colleagues is an example of how genome-wide analysis of DNA methylation levels in AML patients provides valuable information on the relation between DNA methylation and AML disease progression and how methylation profiles correlate with genetic hits [123]. Genome-wide DNA methylation analysis of 344 patients showed the existence of 16 distinct methylation profiles. A number of these profiles correlated with the presence of known translocations like *CBFB-MYH11*, *AML1-ETO*, *PML-RARα* or mutations in *NPM1* or *CEPBα*. Surprisingly, 5 clusters were identified in a group of AMLs that did not share a common translocation or mutation. Most likely, AMLs clustered within these groups share unidentified mutations or deregulated expression of wild type epigenetic modifiers causing deregulated cell cycle control or a block in differentiation. A striking difference in clinical outcome was observed between these different groups, underlining the role of epigenetic regulation in disease progression and the importance of epigenetic analysis as a prognostic tool. The role of epigenetic analysis in survival prediction in AML was emphasized with the identification of a 15 gene methylation classifier which was predictive for clinical outcome in an independent patient cohort.

Most likely, in the near future more genome-wide epigenetic profiling studies on AML samples will be performed, leading to a better understanding of the contributing role of epigenetic hits in AML. As an example, genome-wide occupation analysis of over-expressed epigenetic modifiers like EZH2 and BMI1 and their associated epigenetic modification will be highly informative in elucidating the molecular mechanisms underlying the poor prognosis upon their over-expression. Identification of AML-specific target genes compared to normal hematopoietic cells will inevitably increase our knowledge of the role of epigenetic hits in the process of leukemogenesis, at what stage during disease progression they act and how they collaborate with genetic hits.

Chapter IV

Conclusions

The generation of various genetic models using mouse or human cells has helped tremendously in gaining further insight into the process of leukemic transformation. From these models we have learned how genetic mutations might contribute to the development of hematological malignancies, but also that a single genetic alteration is most often not sufficient to induce overt leukemia. Besides genetic changes, epigenetic alterations, for instance as the consequence of aging, are likely to contribute as well. The challenge in the near future lies in establishing models in which these multiple hits are integrated in order to faithfully recapitulate leukemic development. These models will then provide excellent platforms to study molecular mechanisms involved in leukemic transformation and in which new drug entities can be tested.

References

[1] Passegue E, Jamieson CH, Ailles LE, Weissman IL. Normal and leukemic hematopoiesis: are leukemias a stem cell disorder or a reacquisition of stem cell characteristics? *Proc Natl Acad Sci U S A*. 2003;100 Suppl 111842-11849.

[2] Bonnet D and Dick JE. Human acute myeloid leukemia is organized as a hierarchy that originates from a primitive hematopoietic cell. *Nat Med*. 1997;3(7):730-737.

[3] Hope KJ, Jin L, Dick JE. Acute myeloid leukemia originates from a hierarchy of leukemic stem cell classes that differ in self-renewal capacity. *Nat Immunol*. 2004;5(7):738-743.

[4] Lapidot T, Sirard C, Vormoor J, et al. A cell initiating human acute myeloid leukaemia after transplantation into SCID mice. *Nature*. 1994;367(6464):645-648.

[5] Bhatia M, Wang JC, Kapp U, Bonnet D, Dick JE. Purification of primitive human hematopoietic cells capable of repopulating immune-deficient mice. *Proc Natl Acad Sci U S A*. 1997;94(10):5320-5325.

[6] Taussig DC, Miraki-Moud F, Anjos-Afonso F, et al. Anti-CD38 antibody-mediated clearance of human repopulating cells masks the heterogeneity of leukemia-initiating cells. *Blood*. 2008;112(3):568-575.

[7] Kelly LM and Gilliland DG. Genetics of myeloid leukemias. *Annu Rev Genomics Hum Genet*. 2002;3179-198.

[8] Warner JK, Wang JC, Hope KJ, Jin L, Dick JE. Concepts of human leukemic development. *Oncogene*. 2004;23(43):7164-7177.

[9] Jordan CT and Guzman ML. Mechanisms controlling pathogenesis and survival of leukemic stem cells. *Oncogene.* 2004;23(43):7178-7187.
[10] Link KA, Chou FS, Mulloy JC. Core binding factor at the crossroads: determining the fate of the HSC. *J Cell Physiol.* 2010;222(1):50-56.
[11] Fenske TS, Pengue G, Mathews V, et al. Stem cell expression of the AML1/ETO fusion protein induces a myeloproliferative disorder in mice. *Proc Natl Acad Sci U S A.* 2004;101(42):15184-15189.
[12] Downing JR, Higuchi M, Lenny N, Yeoh AE. Alterations of the AML1 transcription factor in human leukemia. *Semin Cell Dev Biol.* 2000;11(5):347-360.
[13] Higuchi M, O'Brien D, Kumaravelu P, Lenny N, Yeoh EJ, Downing JR. Expression of a conditional AML1-ETO oncogene bypasses embryonic lethality and establishes a murine model of human t(8;21) acute myeloid leukemia. *Cancer Cell.* 2002;1(1):63-74.
[14] de Guzman CG, Warren AJ, Zhang Z, et al. Hematopoietic stem cell expansion and distinct myeloid developmental abnormalities in a murine model of the AML1-ETO translocation. *Mol Cell Biol.* 2002;22(15):5506-5517.
[15] Basecke J, Schwieger M, Griesinger F, et al. AML1/ETO promotes the maintenance of early hematopoietic progenitors in NOD/SCID mice but does not abrogate their lineage specific differentiation. *Leuk Lymphoma.* 2005;46(2):265-272.
[16] Mulloy JC, Cammenga J, MacKenzie KL, Berguido FJ, Moore MA, Nimer SD. The AML1-ETO fusion protein promotes the expansion of human hematopoietic stem cells. *Blood.* 2002;99(1):15-23.
[17] Mulloy JC, Cammenga J, Berguido FJ, et al. Maintaining the self-renewal and differentiation potential of human CD34+ hematopoietic cells using a single genetic element. *Blood.* 2003;102(13):4369-4376.
[18] Balkhi MY, Christopeit M, Chen Y, Geletu M, Behre G. AML1/ETO-induced survivin expression inhibits transcriptional regulation of myeloid differentiation. *Exp Hematol.* 2008;36(11):1449-1460.

[19] Mori H, Colman SM, Xiao Z, et al. Chromosome translocations and covert leukemic clones are generated during normal fetal development. *Proc Natl Acad Sci U S A*. 2002;99(12):8242-8247.
[20] Krejci O, Wunderlich M, Geiger H, et al. p53 signaling in response to increased DNA damage sensitizes AML1-ETO cells to stress-induced death. *Blood*. 2008;111(4):2190-2199.
[21] Kuo YH, Landrette SF, Heilman SA, et al. Cbf beta-SMMHC induces distinct abnormal myeloid progenitors able to develop acute myeloid leukemia. *Cancer Cell*. 2006;9(1):57-68.
[22] Landrette SF, Kuo YH, Hensen K, et al. Plag1 and Plagl2 are oncogenes that induce acute myeloid leukemia in cooperation with Cbfb-MYH11. *Blood*. 2005;105(7):2900-2907.
[23] Wunderlich M, Krejci O, Wei J, Mulloy JC. Human CD34+ cells expressing the inv(16) fusion protein exhibit a myelomonocytic phenotype with greatly enhanced proliferative ability. *Blood*. 2006;108(5):1690-1697.
[24] Turhan AG, Lemoine FM, Debert C, et al. Highly purified primitive hematopoietic stem cells are PML-RARA negative and generate nonclonal progenitors in acute promyelocytic leukemia. *Blood*. 1995;85(8):2154-2161.
[25] Brown D, Kogan S, Lagasse E, et al. A PMLRARalpha transgene initiates murine acute promyelocytic leukemia. *Proc Natl Acad Sci U S A*. 1997;94(6):2551-2556.
[26] Grisolano JL, Wesselschmidt RL, Pelicci PG, Ley TJ. Altered myeloid development and acute leukemia in transgenic mice expressing PML-RAR alpha under control of cathepsin G regulatory sequences. *Blood*. 1997;89(2):376-387.
[27] He LZ, Tribioli C, Rivi R, et al. Acute leukemia with promyelocytic features in PML/RARalpha transgenic mice. *Proc Natl Acad Sci U S A*. 1997;94(10):5302-5307.
[28] Early E, Moore MA, Kakizuka A, et al. Transgenic expression of PML/RARalpha impairs myelopoiesis. *Proc Natl Acad Sci U S A*. 1996;93(15):7900-7904.
[29] Grignani F, Valtieri M, Gabbianelli M, et al. PML/RAR alpha fusion protein expression in normal human hematopoietic progenitors dictates myeloid commitment and the promyelocytic phenotype. *Blood*. 2000;96(4):1531-1537.

[30] Minucci S, Monestiroli S, Giavara S, et al. PML-RAR induces promyelocytic leukemias with high efficiency following retroviral gene transfer into purified murine hematopoietic progenitors. *Blood.* 2002;100(8):2989-2995.

[31] Minucci S, Nervi C, Lo Coco F, Pelicci PG. Histone deacetylases: a common molecular target for differentiation treatment of acute myeloid leukemias? *Oncogene.* 2001;20(24):3110-3115.

[32] Insinga A, Monestiroli S, Ronzoni S, et al. Impairment of p53 acetylation, stability and function by an oncogenic transcription factor. *EMBO J.* 2004;23(5):1144-1154.

[33] Linggi B, Muller-Tidow C, van de Locht L, et al. The t(8;21) fusion protein, AML1 ETO, specifically represses the transcription of the p14(ARF) tumor suppressor in acute myeloid leukemia. *Nat Med.* 2002;8(7):743-750.

[34] Moore MA, Chung KY, Plasilova M, et al. NUP98 dysregulation in myeloid leukemogenesis. *Ann N Y Acad Sci.* 2007;1106114-142.

[35] Kroon E, Thorsteinsdottir U, Mayotte N, Nakamura T, Sauvageau G. NUP98-HOXA9 expression in hemopoietic stem cells induces chronic and acute myeloid leukemias in mice. *EMBO J.* 2001;20(3):350-361.

[36] Chung KY, Morrone G, Schuringa JJ, et al. Enforced expression of NUP98-HOXA9 in human CD34(+) cells enhances stem cell proliferation. *Cancer Res.* 2006;66(24):11781-11791.

[37] Argiropoulos B and Humphries RK. Hox genes in hematopoiesis and leukemogenesis. *Oncogene.* 2007;26(47):6766-6776.

[38] Calvo KR, Sykes DB, Pasillas MP, Kamps MP. Nup98-HoxA9 immortalizes myeloid progenitors, enforces expression of Hoxa9, Hoxa7 and Meis1, and alters cytokine-specific responses in a manner similar to that induced by retroviral co-expression of Hoxa9 and Meis1. *Oncogene.* 2002;21(27):4247-4256.

[39] Wu M, Kwon HY, Rattis F, et al. Imaging hematopoietic precursor division in real time. *Cell Stem Cell.* 2007;1(5):541-554.

[40] Ernst P, Mabon M, Davidson AJ, Zon LI, Korsmeyer SJ. An Mll-dependent Hox program drives hematopoietic progenitor expansion. *Curr Biol.* 2004;14(22):2063-2069.

[41] Lavau C, Szilvassy SJ, Slany R, Cleary ML. Immortalization and leukemic transformation of a myelomonocytic precursor by

retrovirally transduced HRX-ENL. *EMBO J.* 1997;16(14):4226-4237.
[42] Somervaille TC and Cleary ML. Identification and characterization of leukemia stem cells in murine MLL-AF9 acute myeloid leukemia. *Cancer Cell.* 2006;10(4):257-268.
[43] Barabe F, Kennedy JA, Hope KJ, Dick JE. Modeling the initiation and progression of human acute leukemia in mice. *Science.* 2007;316(5824):600-604.
[44] Wei J, Wunderlich M, Fox C, et al. Microenvironment determines lineage fate in a human model of MLL-AF9 leukemia. *Cancer Cell.* 2008;13(6):483-495.
[45] Cozzio A, Passegue E, Ayton PM, Karsunky H, Cleary ML, Weissman IL. Similar MLL-associated leukemias arising from self-renewing stem cells and short-lived myeloid progenitors. *Genes Dev.* 2003;17(24):3029-3035.
[46] Krivtsov AV, Twomey D, Feng Z, et al. Transformation from committed progenitor to leukaemia stem cell initiated by MLL-AF9. *Nature.* 2006;442(7104):818-822.
[47] Chen W, Kumar AR, Hudson WA, et al. Malignant transformation initiated by Mll-AF9: gene dosage and critical target cells. *Cancer Cell.* 2008;13(5):432-440.
[48] Forster A, Pannell R, Drynan LF, et al. Engineering de novo reciprocal chromosomal translocations associated with Mll to replicate primary events of human cancer. *Cancer Cell.* 2003;3(5):449-458.
[49] Kohlmann A, Schoch C, Dugas M, et al. New insights into MLL gene rearranged acute leukemias using gene expression profiling: shared pathways, lineage commitment, and partner genes. *Leukemia.* 2005;19(6):953-964.
[50] Horton SJ, Grier DG, McGonigle GJ, et al. Continuous MLL-ENL expression is necessary to establish a "Hox Code" and maintain immortalization of hematopoietic progenitor cells. *Cancer Res.* 2005;65(20):9245-9252.
[51] Milne TA, Briggs SD, Brock HW, et al. MLL targets SET domain methyltransferase activity to Hox gene promoters. *Mol Cell.* 2002;10(5):1107-1117.
[52] Milne TA, Martin ME, Brock HW, Slany RK, Hess JL. Leukemogenic MLL fusion proteins bind across a broad region of

the Hox a9 locus, promoting transcription and multiple histone modifications. *Cancer Res.* 2005;65(24):11367-11374.
[53] Faber J, Krivtsov AV, Stubbs MC, et al. HOXA9 is required for survival in human MLL-rearranged acute leukemias. *Blood.* 2009;113(11):2375-2385.
[54] Kumar AR, Li Q, Hudson WA, et al. A role for MEIS1 in MLL-fusion gene leukemia. *Blood.* 2009;113(8):1756-1758.
[55] Wong P, Iwasaki M, Somervaille TC, So CW, Cleary ML. Meis1 is an essential and rate-limiting regulator of MLL leukemia stem cell potential. *Genes Dev.* 2007;21(21):2762-2774.
[56] Gishizky ML, Johnson-White J, Witte ON. Efficient transplantation of BCR-ABL-induced chronic myelogenous leukemia-like syndrome in mice. *Proc Natl Acad Sci U S A.* 1993;90(8):3755-3759.
[57] Pear WS, Miller JP, Xu L, et al. Efficient and rapid induction of a chronic myelogenous leukemia-like myeloproliferative disease in mice receiving P210 bcr/abl-transduced bone marrow. *Blood.* 1998;92(10):3780-3792.
[58] Chalandon Y, Jiang X, Christ O, et al. BCR-ABL-transduced human cord blood cells produce abnormal populations in immunodeficient mice. *Leukemia.* 2005;19(3):442-448.
[59] Perez-Caro M, Cobaleda C, Gonzalez-Herrero I, et al. Cancer induction by restriction of oncogene expression to the stem cell compartment. *EMBO J.* 2009;28(1):8-20.
[60] Melo JV and Barnes DJ. Chronic myeloid leukaemia as a model of disease evolution in human cancer. *Nat Rev Cancer.* 2007;7(6):441-453.
[61] Jamieson CH, Ailles LE, Dylla SJ, et al. Granulocyte-macrophage progenitors as candidate leukemic stem cells in blast-crisis CML. *N Engl J Med.* 2004;351(7):657-667.
[62] Fialkow PJ, Singer JW, Raskind WH, et al. Clonal development, stem-cell differentiation, and clinical remissions in acute nonlymphocytic leukemia. *N Engl J Med.* 1987;317(8):468-473.
[63] Takahashi N, Miura I, Saitoh K, Miura AB. Lineage involvement of stem cells bearing the philadelphia chromosome in chronic myeloid leukemia in the chronic phase as shown by a combination of fluorescence-activated cell sorting and fluorescence in situ hybridization. *Blood.* 1998;92(12):4758-4763.

[64] de Groot RP, Raaijmakers JA, Lammers JW, Jove R, Koenderman L. STAT5 activation by BCR-Abl contributes to transformation of K562 leukemia cells. *Blood.* 1999;94(3):1108-1112.

[65] Scherr M, Chaturvedi A, Battmer K, et al. Enhanced sensitivity to inhibition of SHP2, STAT5, and Gab2 expression in chronic myeloid leukemia (CML). *Blood.* 2006;107(8):3279-3287.

[66] Sillaber C, Gesbert F, Frank DA, Sattler M, Griffin JD. STAT5 activation contributes to growth and viability in Bcr/Abl-transformed cells. *Blood.* 2000;95(6):2118-2125.

[67] Ye D, Wolff N, Li L, Zhang S, Ilaria RL, Jr. STAT5 signaling is required for the efficient induction and maintenance of CML in mice. *Blood.* 2006;107(12):4917-4925.

[68] Ren R. Mechanisms of BCR-ABL in the pathogenesis of chronic myelogenous leukaemia. *Nat Rev Cancer.* 2005;5(3):172-183.

[69] Thomas EK, Cancelas JA, Chae HD, et al. Rac guanosine triphosphatases represent integrating molecular therapeutic targets for BCR-ABL-induced myeloproliferative disease. *Cancer Cell.* 2007;12(5):467-478.

[70] Zhao C, Chen A, Jamieson CH, et al. Hedgehog signalling is essential for maintenance of cancer stem cells in myeloid leukaemia. *Nature.* 2009;458(7239):776-779.

[71] Zhang P, Iwasaki-Arai J, Iwasaki H, et al. Enhancement of hematopoietic stem cell repopulating capacity and self-renewal in the absence of the transcription factor C/EBP alpha. *Immunity.* 2004;21(6):853-863.

[72] Barjesteh van Waalwijk van Doorn-Khosrovani, Erpelinck C, Meijer J, et al. Biallelic mutations in the CEBPA gene and low CEBPA expression levels as prognostic markers in intermediate-risk AML. *Hematol J.* 2003;4(1):31-40.

[73] Leroy H, Roumier C, Huyghe P, Biggio V, Fenaux P, Preudhomme C. CEBPA point mutations in hematological malignancies. *Leukemia.* 2005;19(3):329-334.

[74] Kirstetter P, Schuster MB, Bereshchenko O, et al. Modeling of C/EBPalpha mutant acute myeloid leukemia reveals a common expression signature of committed myeloid leukemia-initiating cells. *Cancer Cell.* 2008;13(4):299-310.

[75] Bereshchenko O, Mancini E, Moore S, et al. Hematopoietic stem cell expansion precedes the generation of committed myeloid

leukemia-initiating cells in C/EBPalpha mutant AML. *Cancer Cell.* 2009;16(5):390-400.

[76] Pabst T, Mueller BU, Harakawa N, et al. AML1-ETO downregulates the granulocytic differentiation factor C/EBPalpha in t(8;21) myeloid leukemia. *Nat Med.* 2001;7(4):444-451.

[77] Tenen DG. Abnormalities of the CEBP alpha transcription factor: a major target in acute myeloid leukemia. *Leukemia.* 2001;15(4):688-689.

[78] Lennartsson J, Jelacic T, Linnekin D, Shivakrupa R. Normal and oncogenic forms of the receptor tyrosine kinase kit. *Stem Cells.* 2005;23(1):16-43.

[79] Mackarehtschian K, Hardin JD, Moore KA, Boast S, Goff SP, Lemischka IR. Targeted disruption of the flk2/flt3 gene leads to deficiencies in primitive hematopoietic progenitors. *Immunity.* 1995;3(1):147-161.

[80] Stirewalt DL and Radich JP. The role of FLT3 in haematopoietic malignancies. *Nat Rev Cancer.* 2003;3(9):650-665.

[81] Kelly LM, Liu Q, Kutok JL, Williams IR, Boulton CL, Gilliland DG. FLT3 internal tandem duplication mutations associated with human acute myeloid leukemias induce myeloproliferative disease in a murine bone marrow transplant model. *Blood.* 2002;99(1):310-318.

[82] Li L, Piloto O, Nguyen HB, et al. Knock-in of an internal tandem duplication mutation into murine FLT3 confers myeloproliferative disease in a mouse model. *Blood.* 2008;111(7):3849-3858.

[83] Chung KY, Morrone G, Schuringa JJ, Wong B, Dorn DC, Moore MA. Enforced expression of an Flt3 internal tandem duplication in human CD34+ cells confers properties of self-renewal and enhanced erythropoiesis. *Blood.* 2005;105(1):77-84.

[84] Mizuki M, Fenski R, Halfter H, et al. Flt3 mutations from patients with acute myeloid leukemia induce transformation of 32D cells mediated by the Ras and STAT5 pathways. *Blood.* 2000;96(12):3907-3914.

[85] Rocnik JL, Okabe R, Yu JC, et al. Roles of tyrosine 589 and 591 in STAT5 activation and transformation mediated by FLT3-ITD. *Blood.* 2006;108(4):1339-1345.

[86] Fukuda S, Singh P, Moh A, et al. Survivin mediates aberrant hematopoietic progenitor cell proliferation and acute leukemia in

mice induced by internal tandem duplication of Flt3. *Blood.* 2009;114(2):394-403.

[87] Yoshimoto G, Miyamoto T, Jabbarzadeh-Tabrizi S, et al. FLT3-ITD up-regulates MCL-1 to promote survival of stem cells in acute myeloid leukemia via FLT3-ITD-specific STAT5 activation. *Blood.* 2009;114(24):5034-5043.

[88] Grundler R, Miething C, Thiede C, Peschel C, Duyster J. FLT3-ITD and tyrosine kinase domain mutants induce 2 distinct phenotypes in a murine bone marrow transplantation model. *Blood.* 2005;105(12):4792-4799.

[89] Kitayama H, Tsujimura T, Matsumura I, et al. Neoplastic transformation of normal hematopoietic cells by constitutively activating mutations of c-kit receptor tyrosine kinase. *Blood.* 1996;88(3):995-1004.

[90] Frohling S, Scholl C, Gilliland DG, Levine RL. Genetics of myeloid malignancies: pathogenetic and clinical implications. *J Clin Oncol.* 2005;23(26):6285-6295.

[91] Falini B, Nicoletti I, Bolli N, et al. Translocations and mutations involving the nucleophosmin (NPM1) gene in lymphomas and leukemias. *Haematologica.* 2007;92(4):519-532.

[92] Cheng K, Grisendi S, Clohessy JG, et al. The leukemia-associated cytoplasmic nucleophosmin mutant is an oncogene with paradoxical functions: Arf inactivation and induction of cellular senescence. *Oncogene.* 2007;26(53):7391-7400.

[93] Cheng K, Sportoletti P, Ito K, et al. The cytoplasmic NPM mutant induces myeloproliferation in a transgenic mouse model. *Blood.* 2009.

[94] Tartaglia M, Niemeyer CM, Fragale A, et al. Somatic mutations in PTPN11 in juvenile myelomonocytic leukemia, myelodysplastic syndromes and acute myeloid leukemia. *Nat Genet.* 2003;34(2):148-150.

[95] Bos JL, Rehmann H, Wittinghofer A. GEFs and GAPs: critical elements in the control of small G proteins. *Cell.* 2007;129(5):865-877.

[96] Boguski MS and McCormick F. Proteins regulating Ras and its relatives. *Nature.* 1993;366(6456):643-654.

[97] Parikh C, Subrahmanyam R, Ren R. Oncogenic NRAS, KRAS, and HRAS exhibit different leukemogenic potentials in mice. *Cancer Res.* 2007;67(15):7139-7146.
[98] Shen SW, Dolnikov A, Passioura T, et al. Mutant N-ras preferentially drives human CD34+ hematopoietic progenitor cells into myeloid differentiation and proliferation both in vitro and in the NOD/SCID mouse. *Exp Hematol.* 2004;32(9):852-860.
[99] Braun BS, Tuveson DA, Kong N, et al. Somatic activation of oncogenic Kras in hematopoietic cells initiates a rapidly fatal myeloproliferative disorder. *Proc Natl Acad Sci U S A.* 2004;101(2):597-602.
[100] Chan IT, Kutok JL, Williams IR, et al. Conditional expression of oncogenic K-ras from its endogenous promoter induces a myeloproliferative disease. *J Clin Invest.* 2004;113(4):528-538.
[101] Van Meter ME, Diaz-Flores E, Archard JA, et al. K-RasG12D expression induces hyperproliferation and aberrant signaling in primary hematopoietic stem/progenitor cells. *Blood.* 2007;109(9):3945-3952.
[102] Sabnis AJ, Cheung LS, Dail M, et al. Oncogenic Kras initiates leukemia in hematopoietic stem cells. *PLoS Biol.* 2009;7(3):e59.
[103] Zhang J, Wang J, Liu Y, et al. Oncogenic Kras-induced leukemogeneis: hematopoietic stem cells as the initial target and lineage-specific progenitors as the potential targets for final leukemic transformation. *Blood.* 2009;113(6):1304-1314.
[104] Alvarado Y and Giles FJ. Ras as a therapeutic target in hematologic malignancies. *Expert Opin Emerg Drugs.* 2007;12(2):271-284.
[105] Scholl C, Gilliland DG, Frohling S. Deregulation of signaling pathways in acute myeloid leukemia. *Semin Oncol.* 2008;35(4):336-345.
[106] Goldberg AD, Allis CD, Bernstein E. Epigenetics: a landscape takes shape. *Cell.* 2007;128(4):635-638.
[107] Berger SL, Kouzarides T, Shiekhattar R, Shilatifard A. An operational definition of epigenetics. *Genes Dev.* 2009;23(7):781-783.
[108] Kouzarides T. Chromatin modifications and their function. *Cell.* 2007;128(4):693-705.

[109] Bird A. DNA methylation patterns and epigenetic memory. *Genes Dev.* 2002;16(1):6-21.
[110] Jones PL, Veenstra GJ, Wade PA, et al. Methylated DNA and MeCP2 recruit histone deacetylase to repress transcription. *Nat Genet.* 1998;19(2):187-191.
[111] Suzuki MM and Bird A. DNA methylation landscapes: provocative insights from epigenomics. *Nat Rev Genet.* 2008;9(6):465-476.
[112] Weber M and Schubeler D. Genomic patterns of DNA methylation: targets and function of an epigenetic mark. *Curr Opin Cell Biol.* 2007;19(3):273-280.
[113] Ting AH, McGarvey KM, Baylin SB. The cancer epigenome-- components and functional correlates. *Genes Dev.* 2006;20(23):3215-3231.
[114] Jones PA and Baylin SB. The epigenomics of cancer. *Cell.* 2007;128(4):683-692.
[115] Claus R and Lubbert M. Epigenetic targets in hematopoietic malignancies. *Oncogene.* 2003;22(42):6489-6496.
[116] Herman JG, Civin CI, Issa JP, Collector MI, Sharkis SJ, Baylin SB. Distinct patterns of inactivation of p15INK4B and p16INK4A characterize the major types of hematological malignancies. *Cancer Res.* 1997;57(5):837-841.
[117] Kim WY and Sharpless NE. The regulation of INK4/ARF in cancer and aging. *Cell.* 2006;127(2):265-275.
[118] Uchida T, Kinoshita T, Nagai H, et al. Hypermethylation of the p15INK4B gene in myelodysplastic syndromes. *Blood.* 1997;90(4):1403-1409.
[119] Agrawal S, Unterberg M, Koschmieder S, et al. DNA methylation of tumor suppressor genes in clinical remission predicts the relapse risk in acute myeloid leukemia. *Cancer Res.* 2007;67(3):1370-1377.
[120] Latres E, Malumbres M, Sotillo R, et al. Limited overlapping roles of P15(INK4b) and P18(INK4c) cell cycle inhibitors in proliferation and tumorigenesis. *EMBO J.* 2000;19(13):3496-3506.
[121] Wolff L, Garin MT, Koller R, et al. Hypermethylation of the Ink4b locus in murine myeloid leukemia and increased susceptibility to leukemia in p15(Ink4b)-deficient mice. *Oncogene.* 2003;22(58):9265-9274.

[122] Kroeger H, Jelinek J, Estecio MR, et al. Aberrant CpG island methylation in acute myeloid leukemia is accentuated at relapse. *Blood.* 2008;112(4):1366-1373.
[123] Figueroa ME, Lugthart S, Li Y, et al. DNA Methylation Signatures Identify Biologically Distinct Subtypes in Acute Myeloid Leukemia. *Cancer Cell.* 2010.
[124] Daskalakis M, Nguyen TT, Nguyen C, et al. Demethylation of a hypermethylated P15/INK4B gene in patients with myelodysplastic syndrome by 5-Aza-2'-deoxycytidine (decitabine) treatment. *Blood.* 2002;100(8):2957-2964.
[125] Garcia-Manero G. Demethylating agents in myeloid malignancies. *Curr Opin Oncol.* 2008;20(6):705-710.
[126] Borrow J, Stanton VP, Jr., Andresen JM, et al. The translocation t(8;16)(p11;p13) of acute myeloid leukaemia fuses a putative acetyltransferase to the CREB-binding protein. *Nat Genet.* 1996;14(1):33-41.
[127] Chaffanet M, Gressin L, Preudhomme C, Soenen-Cornu V, Birnbaum D, Pebusque MJ. MOZ is fused to p300 in an acute monocytic leukemia with t(8;22). *Genes Chromosomes Cancer.* 2000;28(2):138-144.
[128] Kitabayashi I, Aikawa Y, Yokoyama A, et al. Fusion of MOZ and p300 histone acetyltransferases in acute monocytic leukemia with a t(8;22)(p11;q13) chromosome translocation. *Leukemia.* 2001;15(1):89-94.
[129] Carapeti M, Aguiar RC, Goldman JM, Cross NC. A novel fusion between MOZ and the nuclear receptor coactivator TIF2 in acute myeloid leukemia. *Blood.* 1998;91(9):3127-3133.
[130] Liang J, Prouty L, Williams BJ, Dayton MA, Blanchard KL. Acute mixed lineage leukemia with an inv(8)(p11q13) resulting in fusion of the genes for MOZ and TIF2. *Blood.* 1998;92(6):2118-2122.
[131] Esteyries S, Perot C, Adelaide J, et al. NCOA3, a new fusion partner for MOZ/MYST3 in M5 acute myeloid leukemia. *Leukemia.* 2008;22(3):663-665.
[132] Kojima K, Kaneda K, Yoshida C, et al. A novel fusion variant of the MORF and CBP genes detected in therapy-related myelodysplastic syndrome with t(10;16)(q22;p13). *Br J Haematol.* 2003;120(2):271-273.

[133] Panagopoulos I, Fioretos T, Isaksson M, et al. Fusion of the MORF and CBP genes in acute myeloid leukemia with the t(10;16)(q22;p13). *Hum Mol Genet.* 2001;10(4):395-404.

[134] Deguchi K, Ayton PM, Carapeti M, et al. MOZ-TIF2-induced acute myeloid leukemia requires the MOZ nucleosome binding motif and TIF2-mediated recruitment of CBP. *Cancer Cell.* 2003;3(3):259-271.

[135] Collins HM, Kindle KB, Matsuda S, et al. MOZ-TIF2 alters cofactor recruitment and histone modification at the RARbeta2 promoter: differential effects of MOZ fusion proteins on CBP- and MOZ-dependent activators. *J Biol Chem.* 2006;281(25):17124-17133.

[136] Kindle KB, Troke PJ, Collins HM, et al. MOZ-TIF2 inhibits transcription by nuclear receptors and p53 by impairment of CBP function. *Mol Cell Biol.* 2005;25(3):988-1002.

[137] Thomas T, Corcoran LM, Gugasyan R, et al. Monocytic leukemia zinc finger protein is essential for the development of long-term reconstituting hematopoietic stem cells. *Genes Dev.* 2006;20(9):1175-1186.

[138] Perez-Campo FM, Borrow J, Kouskoff V, Lacaud G. The histone acetyl transferase activity of monocytic leukemia zinc finger is critical for the proliferation of hematopoietic precursors. *Blood.* 2009;113(20):4866-4874.

[139] Camos M, Esteve J, Jares P, et al. Gene expression profiling of acute myeloid leukemia with translocation t(8;16)(p11;p13) and MYST3-CREBBP rearrangement reveals a distinctive signature with a specific pattern of HOX gene expression. *Cancer Res.* 2006;66(14):6947-6954.

[140] Crump JG, Swartz ME, Eberhart JK, Kimmel CB. Moz-dependent Hox expression controls segment-specific fate maps of skeletal precursors in the face. *Development.* 2006;133(14):2661-2669.

[141] Miller CT, Maves L, Kimmel CB. moz regulates Hox expression and pharyngeal segmental identity in zebrafish. *Development.* 2004;131(10):2443-2461.

[142] Voss AK, Collin C, Dixon MP, Thomas T. Moz and retinoic acid coordinately regulate H3K9 acetylation, Hox gene expression, and segment identity. *Dev Cell.* 2009;17(5):674-686.

[143] Schuettengruber B, Chourrout D, Vervoort M, Leblanc B, Cavalli G. Genome regulation by polycomb and trithorax proteins. *Cell.* 2007;128(4):735-745.
[144] Nakamura T, Mori T, Tada S, et al. ALL-1 is a histone methyltransferase that assembles a supercomplex of proteins involved in transcriptional regulation. *Mol Cell.* 2002;10(5):1119-1128.
[145] Hess JL, Yu BD, Li B, Hanson R, Korsmeyer SJ. Defects in yolk sac hematopoiesis in Mll-null embryos. *Blood.* 1997;90(5):1799-1806.
[146] Ernst P, Fisher JK, Avery W, Wade S, Foy D, Korsmeyer SJ. Definitive hematopoiesis requires the mixed-lineage leukemia gene. *Dev Cell.* 2004;6(3):437-443.
[147] Jude CD, Climer L, Xu D, Artinger E, Fisher JK, Ernst P. Unique and independent roles for MLL in adult hematopoietic stem cells and progenitors. *Cell Stem Cell.* 2007;1(3):324-337.
[148] McMahon KA, Hiew SY, Hadjur S, et al. Mll has a critical role in fetal and adult hematopoietic stem cell self-renewal. *Cell Stem Cell.* 2007;1(3):338-345.
[149] Krivtsov AV and Armstrong SA. MLL translocations, histone modifications and leukaemia stem-cell development. *Nat Rev Cancer.* 2007;7(11):823-833.
[150] Krivtsov AV, Feng Z, Lemieux ME, et al. H3K79 methylation profiles define murine and human MLL-AF4 leukemias. *Cancer Cell.* 2008;14(5):355-368.
[151] Okada Y, Feng Q, Lin Y, et al. hDOT1L links histone methylation to leukemogenesis. *Cell.* 2005;121(2):167-178.
[152] Guenther MG, Lawton LN, Rozovskaia T, et al. Aberrant chromatin at genes encoding stem cell regulators in human mixed-lineage leukemia. *Genes Dev.* 2008;22(24):3403-3408.
[153] Shi Y and Whetstine JR. Dynamic regulation of histone lysine methylation by demethylases. *Mol Cell.* 2007;25(1):1-14.
[154] van Zutven LJ, Onen E, Velthuizen SC, et al. Identification of NUP98 abnormalities in acute leukemia: JARID1A (12p13) as a new partner gene. *Genes Chromosomes Cancer.* 2006;45(5):437-446.

[155] Wang GG, Song J, Wang Z, et al. Haematopoietic malignancies caused by dysregulation of a chromatin-binding PHD finger. *Nature*. 2009;459(7248):847-851.
[156] Schwartz YB and Pirrotta V. Polycomb silencing mechanisms and the management of genomic programmes. *Nat Rev Genet*. 2007;8(1):9-22.
[157] Cao R, Wang L, Wang H, et al. Role of histone H3 lysine 27 methylation in Polycomb-group silencing. *Science*. 2002;298(5595):1039-1043.
[158] Cao R and Zhang Y. The functions of E(Z)/EZH2-mediated methylation of lysine 27 in histone H3. *Curr Opin Genet Dev*. 2004;14(2):155-164.
[159] Dellino GI, Schwartz YB, Farkas G, McCabe D, Elgin SC, Pirrotta V. Polycomb silencing blocks transcription initiation. *Mol Cell*. 2004;13(6):887-893.
[160] Shao Z, Raible F, Mollaaghababa R, et al. Stabilization of chromatin structure by PRC1, a Polycomb complex. *Cell*. 1999;98(1):37-46.
[161] Wang H, Wang L, Erdjument-Bromage H, et al. Role of histone H2A ubiquitination in Polycomb silencing. *Nature*. 2004;431(7010):873-878.
[162] de NM, Mermoud JE, Wakao R, et al. Polycomb group proteins Ring1A/B link ubiquitylation of histone H2A to heritable gene silencing and X inactivation. *Dev Cell*. 2004;7(5):663-676.
[163] Cao R, Tsukada Y, Zhang Y. Role of Bmi-1 and Ring1A in H2A ubiquitylation and Hox gene silencing. *Mol Cell*. 2005;20(6):845-854.
[164] Kallin EM, Cao R, Jothi R, et al. Genome-wide uH2A localization analysis highlights Bmi1-dependent deposition of the mark at repressed genes. *PLoS Genet*. 2009;5(6):e1000506.
[165] Boyer LA, Plath K, Zeitlinger J, et al. Polycomb complexes repress developmental regulators in murine embryonic stem cells. *Nature*. 2006;441(7091):349-353.
[166] Lee TI, Jenner RG, Boyer LA, et al. Control of developmental regulators by Polycomb in human embryonic stem cells. *Cell*. 2006;125(2):301-313.

[167] Bracken AP, Dietrich N, Pasini D, Hansen KH, Helin K. Genome-wide mapping of Polycomb target genes unravels their roles in cell fate transitions. *Genes Dev.* 2006;20(9):1123-1136.
[168] Varambally S, Dhanasekaran SM, Zhou M, et al. The polycomb group protein EZH2 is involved in progression of prostate cancer. *Nature.* 2002;419(6907):624-629.
[169] Kleer CG, Cao Q, Varambally S, et al. EZH2 is a marker of aggressive breast cancer and promotes neoplastic transformation of breast epithelial cells. *Proc Natl Acad Sci U S A.* 2003;100(20):11606-11611.
[170] Bracken AP, Pasini D, Capra M, Prosperini E, Colli E, Helin K. EZH2 is downstream of the pRB-E2F pathway, essential for proliferation and amplified in cancer. *EMBO J.* 2003;22(20):5323-5335.
[171] Kamminga LM, Bystrykh LV, de BA, et al. The Polycomb group gene Ezh2 prevents hematopoietic stem cell exhaustion. *Blood.* 2006;107(5):2170-2179.
[172] Villa R, Pasini D, Gutierrez A, et al. Role of the polycomb repressive complex 2 in acute promyelocytic leukemia. *Cancer Cell.* 2007;11(6):513-525.
[173] Sawa M, Yamamoto K, Yokozawa T, et al. BMI-1 is highly expressed in M0-subtype acute myeloid leukemia. *Int J Hematol.* 2005;82(1):42-47.
[174] Bea S, Tort F, Pinyol M, et al. BMI-1 gene amplification and overexpression in hematological malignancies occur mainly in mantle cell lymphomas. *Cancer Res.* 2001;61(6):2409-2412.
[175] Chowdhury M, Mihara K, Yasunaga S, Ohtaki M, Takihara Y, Kimura A. Expression of Polycomb-group (PcG) protein BMI-1 predicts prognosis in patients with acute myeloid leukemia. *Leukemia.* 2007;21(5):1116-1122.
[176] Haupt Y, Alexander WS, Barri G, Klinken SP, Adams JM. Novel zinc finger gene implicated as myc collaborator by retrovirally accelerated lymphomagenesis in E mu-myc transgenic mice. *Cell.* 1991;65(5):753-763.
[177] van LM, Verbeek S, Scheijen B, Wientjens E, van der GH, Berns A. Identification of cooperating oncogenes in E mu-myc transgenic mice by provirus tagging. *Cell.* 1991;65(5):737-752.

[178] van der Lugt NM, Domen J, Linders K, et al. Posterior transformation, neurological abnormalities, and severe hematopoietic defects in mice with a targeted deletion of the bmi-1 proto-oncogene. *Genes Dev.* 1994;8(7):757-769.

[179] Park IK, Qian D, Kiel M, et al. Bmi-1 is required for maintenance of adult self-renewing haematopoietic stem cells. *Nature.* 2003;423(6937):302-305.

[180] Iwama A, Oguro H, Negishi M, et al. Enhanced self-renewal of hematopoietic stem cells mediated by the polycomb gene product Bmi-1. *Immunity.* 2004;21(6):843-851.

[181] Lessard J and Sauvageau G. Bmi-1 determines the proliferative capacity of normal and leukaemic stem cells. *Nature.* 2003;423(6937):255-260.

[182] Rizo A, Dontje B, Vellenga E, de HG, Schuringa JJ. Long-term maintenance of human hematopoietic stem/progenitor cells by expression of BMI1. *Blood.* 2008;111(5):2621-2630.

[183] Rizo A, Olthof S, Han L, Vellenga E, de HG, Schuringa JJ. Repression of BMI1 in normal and leukemic human CD34(+) cells impairs self-renewal and induces apoptosis. *Blood.* 2009;114(8):1498-1505.

[184] Jacobs JJ, Kieboom K, Marino S, DePinho RA, van LM. The oncogene and Polycomb-group gene bmi-1 regulates cell proliferation and senescence through the ink4a locus. *Nature.* 1999;397(6715):164-168.

[185] Bruggeman SW, Valk-Lingbeek ME, van der Stoop PP, et al. Ink4a and Arf differentially affect cell proliferation and neural stem cell self-renewal in Bmi1-deficient mice. *Genes Dev.* 2005;19(12):1438-1443.

[186] Liu J, Cao L, Chen J, et al. Bmi1 regulates mitochondrial function and the DNA damage response pathway. *Nature.* 2009;459(7245):387-392.

[187] Dash A and Gilliland DG. Molecular genetics of acute myeloid leukaemia. *Best Pract Res Clin Haematol.* 2001;14(1):49-64.

[188] Chan IT, Kutok JL, Williams IR, et al. Oncogenic K-ras cooperates with PML-RAR alpha to induce an acute promyelocytic leukemia-like disease. *Blood.* 2006;108(5):1708-1715.

[189] Kelly LM, Kutok JL, Williams IR, et al. PML/RARalpha and FLT3-ITD induce an APL-like disease in a mouse model. *Proc Natl Acad Sci U S A*. 2002;99(12):8283-8288.
[190] Schessl C, Rawat VP, Cusan M, et al. The AML1-ETO fusion gene and the FLT3 length mutation collaborate in inducing acute leukemia in mice. *J Clin Invest*. 2005;115(8):2159-2168.
[191] Zheng X, Oancea C, Henschler R, Ruthardt M. Cooperation between constitutively activated c-Kit signaling and leukemogenic transcription factors in the determination of the leukemic phenotype in murine hematopoietic stem cells. *Int J Oncol*. 2009;34(6):1521-1531.
[192] Suzuki T, Kiyoi H, Ozeki K, et al. Clinical characteristics and prognostic implications of NPM1 mutations in acute myeloid leukemia. *Blood*. 2005;106(8):2854-2861.
[193] Boukarabila H, Saurin AJ, Batsche E, et al. The PRC1 Polycomb group complex interacts with PLZF/RARA to mediate leukemic transformation. *Genes Dev*. 2009;23(10):1195-1206.
[194] Yergeau DA, Hetherington CJ, Wang Q, et al. Embryonic lethality and impairment of haematopoiesis in mice heterozygous for an AML1-ETO fusion gene. *Nat Genet*. 1997;15(3):303-306.
[195] Castilla LH, Wijmenga C, Wang Q, et al. Failure of embryonic hematopoiesis and lethal hemorrhages in mouse embryos heterozygous for a knocked-in leukemia gene CBFB-MYH11. *Cell*. 1996;87(4):687-696.
[196] Castilla LH, Garrett L, Adya N, et al. The fusion gene Cbfb-MYH11 blocks myeloid differentiation and predisposes mice to acute myelomonocytic leukaemia. *Nat Genet*. 1999;23(2):144-146.
[197] Iwasaki M, Kuwata T, Yamazaki Y, et al. Identification of cooperative genes for NUP98-HOXA9 in myeloid leukemogenesis using a mouse model. *Blood*. 2005;105(2):784-793.
[198] Corral J, Lavenir I, Impey H, et al. An Mll-AF9 fusion gene made by homologous recombination causes acute leukemia in chimeric mice: a method to create fusion oncogenes. *Cell*. 1996;85(6):853-861.
[199] Dobson CL, Warren AJ, Pannell R, et al. The mll-AF9 gene fusion in mice controls myeloproliferation and specifies acute myeloid leukaemogenesis. *EMBO J*. 1999;18(13):3564-3574.

[200] Honda H, Fujii T, Takatoku M, et al. Expression of p210bcr/abl by metallothionein promoter induced T-cell leukemia in transgenic mice. *Blood*. 1995;85(10):2853-2861.

[201] Voncken JW, Kaartinen V, Pattengale PK, Germeraad WT, Groffen J, Heisterkamp N. BCR/ABL P210 and P190 cause distinct leukemia in transgenic mice. *Blood*. 1995;86(12):4603-4611.

[202] Honda H, Oda H, Suzuki T, et al. Development of acute lymphoblastic leukemia and myeloproliferative disorder in transgenic mice expressing p210bcr/abl: a novel transgenic model for human Ph1-positive leukemias. *Blood*. 1998;91(6):2067-2075.

[203] Huettner CS, Zhang P, Van Etten RA, Tenen DG. Reversibility of acute B-cell leukaemia induced by BCR-ABL1. *Nat Genet*. 2000;24(1):57-60.

[204] Chalandon Y, Jiang X, Hazlewood G, et al. Modulation of p210(BCR-ABL) activity in transduced primary human hematopoietic cells controls lineage programming. *Blood*. 2002;99(9):3197-3204.

[205] Schwieger M, Lohler J, Fischer M, Herwig U, Tenen DG, Stocking C. A dominant-negative mutant of C/EBPalpha, associated with acute myeloid leukemias, inhibits differentiation of myeloid and erythroid progenitors of man but not mouse. *Blood*. 2004;103(7):2744-2752.

Index

A

acid, 4, 8, 42
acute leukemia, 3, 6, 10, 25, 33, 34, 35, 38, 43, 46, 47
acute lymphoblastic leukemia, 47
acute myeloid leukemia, 18, 31, 32, 33, 34, 37, 38, 39, 40, 41, 42, 45, 46, 47
acute nonlymphocytic leukemia, 36
acute promyelocytic leukemia, 5, 33, 45, 46
allele, 8, 12
alters, 34, 42
antibody, 31
antioxidant, 24
APL, 5, 8, 25, 46
apoptosis, 11, 24, 46
arginine, 21

B

binding, 3, 8, 13, 18, 23, 32, 41, 42, 43
birth, 11, 13
blood, 1, 4, 10, 11, 14, 15, 24, 36
BMI, 45
bone, vii, 4, 15, 20, 22, 26, 35, 38
bone marrow, vii, 4, 15, 20, 22, 26, 35, 38
bone marrow transplant, 20, 38
breast cancer, 44

C

cancer, vii, 18, 19, 23, 35, 36, 37, 40, 44
cancer cells, 18, 19
cathepsin G, 33
cell, vii, 1, 2, 6, 7, 9, 10, 15, 17, 19, 22, 23, 25, 26, 27, 31, 32, 34, 35, 36, 37, 38, 41, 43, 44, 45, 46, 47
cell cycle, 24, 27, 41
cell death, 24
cell fate, vii, 44
cell line, 10, 19, 22
cell lines, 10
centrosome, 14
chemotherapy, 8
chimera, 5
chromosome, 17, 36, 41
chronic myelogenous, 35, 36
classes, 31
clone, 1, 4
combined effect, 13
components, 23, 40
control, 27, 33, 39
CSF, 9
cytoplasm, 14
cytosine, 18

D

defects, 2, 21, 45
deficiencies, 37
definition, 17, 40
delivery, 4, 8, 10, 14
differentiation, v, vii, 1, 2, 3, 5, 6, 7, 8, 9, 11, 13, 15, 17, 21, 25, 26, 27, 32, 33, 36, 37, 39, 47
disease progression, 12, 19, 23, 26, 27
diseases, 23
disorder, 1, 3, 5, 6, 7, 9, 13, 15, 31, 32, 39, 47
division, 9, 23, 34
DNA, 3, 4, 13, 17, 19, 24, 26, 32, 40, 41, 46
DNA damage, 24, 32, 46
DNA repair, 4, 26
dosage, 7, 35
down-regulation, 22
Drosophila, 21, 22
duplication, 14, 37, 38

E

embryonic stem cells, 44
encoding, 3, 21, 43
engineering, 13
enzymes, 17, 26
epigenetics, 17, 40
epithelial cells, 44
euchromatin, 17
evolution, 36

F

family, 20, 21, 22
fetal development, 32
fusion, 3, 4, 8, 9, 10, 11, 13, 14, 15, 20, 21, 22, 23, 32, 33, 35, 41, 42, 46, 47

G

GDP, 15
gene, 3, 8, 9, 10, 11, 13, 14, 17, 18, 19, 20, 21, 23, 26, 27, 33, 35, 37, 38, 40, 41, 42, 43, 44, 45, 46, 47
gene amplification, 45
gene expression, 17, 18, 20, 21, 22, 26, 35, 42
gene promoter, 13, 23, 35
gene silencing, 44
gene targeting, 3
gene transfer, 33
generation, 4, 11, 18, 29, 37
genes, 3, 4, 8, 9, 10, 11, 12, 14, 15, 17, 18, 19, 20, 21, 22, 23, 24, 26, 27, 34, 35, 40, 41, 42, 43, 44, 47
genetic alteration, 17, 29
genetic defect, 1
genetic mutations, 26, 29
genetics, 46
genome, 18, 19, 22, 26, 27
genomic instability, 11
genotype, 17
groups, 12, 18, 19, 27
growth, 7, 11, 14, 19, 36
growth factor, 14

H

hematopoietic development, 10
hematopoietic stem cells, vii, 26, 32, 33, 39, 42, 43, 45, 46
hematopoietic system, 1
heterochromatin, 17
heterogeneity, 1, 31
histone, 8, 17, 20, 21, 22, 23, 35, 40, 41, 42, 43, 44
hydrolysis, 15
hyperplasia, 19
hypothesis, vii, 25

Index

I

identification, 22, 27
in situ hybridization, 36
in vitro, 4, 5, 6, 7, 9, 11, 39
in vivo, 4, 6, 7, 9
incidence, 2, 11, 25
independence, 14
induction, 12, 24, 35, 36, 39
inhibition, 8, 18, 36
inhibitor, 23
initiation, 12, 18, 19, 21, 23, 34, 44
insight, 13, 29
interactions, 26
interphase, 17

J

Jordan, 31

K

karyotype, 14
kinetics, 7

L

landscape, 26, 40
landscapes, 26, 40
latency, 5, 6, 7, 8, 9, 10, 11, 13, 25
leukemia, vii, 1, 2, 4, 5, 6, 7, 8, 9, 10, 13, 14, 15, 17, 19, 21, 22, 25, 29, 31, 32, 33, 34, 35, 36, 37, 38, 39, 41, 42, 43, 47
liver, 5, 13, 24
liver cells, 13, 24
localization, 12, 14, 23, 44
locus, 13, 24, 35, 41, 46
lymph node, 19
lymphoid, 5, 6, 10, 11, 14, 19
lymphoma, 6, 7, 14, 15
lysine, 20, 21, 22, 23, 43, 44

M

maintenance, 1, 3, 11, 18, 20, 21, 32, 36, 37, 45
majority, 8, 11, 18
malignancy, 15
maturation, 1
Mayotte, 34
metabolism, 24
methylation, 17, 19, 21, 22, 26, 40, 41, 43, 44
mice, 3, 4, 5, 6, 7, 8, 10, 11, 13, 14, 15, 19, 20, 21, 23, 25, 31, 32, 33, 34, 35, 36, 38, 39, 41, 45, 46, 47
migration, 1
model, 3, 4, 8, 10, 11, 13, 14, 15, 18, 22, 24, 25, 32, 34, 36, 38, 39, 46, 47
model system, 24
modeling, 11
models, 3, 5, 9, 11, 12, 13, 14, 15, 19, 21, 23, 25, 29
multipotent, 1
mutagen, 4
mutagenesis, 8
mutant, 7, 13, 14, 15, 37, 38, 39, 47
mutation, 4, 12, 15, 25, 27, 38, 46
mutation rate, 4
myelodysplastic syndromes, 39, 40
myeloid cells, 4, 5, 8, 13

N

nuclear receptors, 20, 42
nuclei, 17
nucleosome, 17, 42
nucleus, 14

O

oncogenes, 2, 18, 33, 45, 47
oxidative stress, 26
oxygen, 24

P

pathogenesis, 31, 36
pathways, 4, 18, 24, 26, 35, 38
penetrance, 5, 6, 7, 8, 10, 14, 15
phenotype, 10, 13, 14, 17, 21, 23, 24, 33, 46
phosphorylation, 17
point mutation, 12, 15, 20, 37
polymerase, 23
poor, 13, 23, 27
population, vii, 1, 13
prediction, 27
prevention, 22
prognosis, 13, 23, 27, 45
program, 34
programming, 47
proliferation, 1, 4, 5, 6, 7, 9, 10, 11, 12, 13, 15, 26, 34, 38, 39, 41, 42, 44, 46
promoter, 3, 8, 10, 11, 14, 15, 18, 19, 39, 42, 47
properties, 1, 2, 26, 38
prostate, 23, 44
prostate cancer, 44
proteins, 3, 10, 11, 13, 15, 18, 21, 22, 35, 39, 42, 43, 44
proto-oncogene, 45

R

reactive oxygen, 24
receptors, 2, 13
reciprocal translocation, 11
recombination, 10, 47
recovery, 24
recruiting, 22, 26
regulation, 1, 4, 13, 17, 18, 19, 20, 22, 24, 26, 27, 32, 40, 43
regulators, 43, 44
remission, 8, 19, 40
repression, 8, 18, 21, 23
residues, 17, 20, 21
retrovirus, 19
ribosome, 14
risk, 19, 37, 40
RNA, 23
RNAi, 24

S

senescence, 24, 39, 46
sensitivity, 36
shape, 40
signal transduction, 2
signaling pathway, 12, 15, 40
signalling, 37
solid tumors, 19
spleen, 19
stability, 33
stem cells, vii, 1, 19, 31, 34, 36, 37, 38, 45
stress, 8, 23, 24, 32
survival, 8, 13, 15, 19, 23, 25, 26, 27, 31, 35, 38
susceptibility, 41
symmetry, 26
syndrome, 9, 19, 35, 41, 42

T

T cell, 7, 14, 15
targets, 18, 35, 39, 40
therapeutic targets, 36
therapy, 42
transcription, 3, 9, 12, 14, 18, 19, 22, 32, 33, 35, 37, 40, 42, 44, 46
transcription factors, 18, 22, 46
transduction, 5, 6, 7, 8, 9, 10, 11, 26
transformation, vii, 2, 20, 26, 29, 34, 35, 36, 38, 39, 44, 45, 46
transgene, 33
transition, 4, 12
translocation, 3, 4, 9, 10, 11, 20, 22, 26, 27, 32, 41, 42
transplantation, 1, 4, 6, 8, 10, 11, 15, 20, 23, 24, 26, 31, 35

tumor, 14, 18, 19, 21, 23, 34, 40
tumorigenesis, 41
tumors, 23
tyrosine, 2, 11, 13, 37, 38

Z

zinc, 42, 45

W

wild type, 27